Health Professions Admissions Guide:
Strategy for Success

CO-EDITORS

Carol Baffi-Dugan
Robert E. Cannon

CONTRIBUTORS

Carol Baffi-Dugan

Robert Cannon

Jane Crawford

Paul Crosby

Glenn Cummings

Karen deOlivares

Cecilia Fox

Julian Frankenberg

John Friede

William Hussey

Debra Kirchhof-Glazier

John Klein

Cynthia Lewis

Zelda Lipman

Ronald McCune

Lee Ann Michelson

James Nielsen

Sally Olexia

Kirsten Peterson

Helen Pigage

Norman Sansing

Laurence Savett

Alice Sima

Anthony Smulders

Consuelo Lopez Springfield

Marliss Strange

Edward Trachtenberg

Peter Van Houten

SPECIAL RECOGNITION

Brice Corder
Editor of the first four editions

NAAHP

National Association of Advisors for the Health Professions, Inc.
P.O. Box 1518
Champaign, Illinois 61824-1518
phone: (217) 355-0063   fax: (217) 355-1287   email: naahpinc@aol.com
www.NAAHP.org

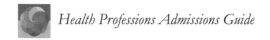
Health Professions Admissions Guide: Strategy for Success

Eighth Edition

Copyright 1990, 1992, 1994, 1998, 2001, 2004, 2007, 2009 by the National Association of Advisors for the Health Professions, Inc.

Special discounts on bulk quantities of NAAHP books are available to NAAHP members, professional associations, and other organizations. For details, contact NAAHP, Inc., P.O. Box 1518, Champaign, IL 61824-1518. Tel: 217-355-0063 Fax: 217-355-1287 www.NAAHP.org

Printed in the United States of America

Published by the National Association of Advisors for the Health Professions, Inc.

Library of Congress Cataloging-in-Publication Data

Health Professions Admissions Guide: Strategy for Success / editors, Carol Baffi-Dugan and Robert Cannon, contributors, Jane Crawford. . . (et al.).

p.cm.

Includes bibliographic references.

ISBN 0-911899-14-6: $22.00
1. Medicine - Vocational guidance - United States - Handbooks, manuals, etc.
2. Allied health personnel - Vocational guidance - United States — Handbooks, manuals, etc.
3. Medical education — United States — Handbooks, manuals, etc.
    I.   Baffi-Dugan, Carol.
    II. National Association of Advisors for the Health Professions.

RC90.S77 2001

610'.69'0973-dc20   90-32510

                                                                                CIP

Production Editor: Kristen Cota
Cover Design: Kristen Cota
Printing and Binding: Premier Print Group

ISBN 978-0-911899-17-7

Table of Contents

PREFACE

The National Association of Advisors for the Health Professions, Inc. (NAAHP), is an organization of approximately one thousand health professions advisors at colleges and universities throughout the United States as well as a few hundred health professions schools and associations. The strength and success of NAAHP is derived from its four regional associations, Central (CAAHP), Northeast (NEAAHP), Southeastern (SAAHP), and Western (WAAHP). Established in 1974, NAAHP is the only national organization concerned exclusively with the needs of health professions advisors and their students. The organization serves as a resource for the professional development of health professions advisors, health professions schools, and professional school associations. It is a representative voice with health professions schools and their professional associations, undergraduate institutions and other health professions organizations. The Association promotes high standards for health professions advising at universities and colleges. The Association assists advisors in fostering the intellectual, personal, and humanistic development of students who are preparing for careers in the health professions. In addition, NAAHP has become an important liaison with health professions institutions, many of whom are patron members of the Association. In its continuing enterprise to serve advisors and prehealth professions students, NAAHP is pleased to offer the eighth edition of this guide.

Whether you are firmly committed to a career in one of the recognized health professions, or simply wish to know more about what is required for pursuing various health care careers, this guide is for you. Further, while this publication is intended primarily for students enrolled in two-year and four-year colleges and universities, the importance of the high school years is also recognized.

As you contemplate a career in one of the health professions, be mindful that many factors will contribute to your success, but none will be more important than obtaining accurate health career and health professions school information. Take advantage of the advising services available at your institution. Most colleges and universities have an office or individual who specializes in providing health professions advice and information. This person is commonly known as the "health professions advisor" or "premedical advisor" even though s/he may be a career advisor for all of the health professions. It is to your benefit to seek out this office and become acquainted with the person to whom you can go for information and advice. As you read through this guide you will notice it is frequently suggested that you speak with your health professions advisor about matters beyond the scope of this publication. This recommendation is probably the best advice we can give. The editors view this publication as a supplement; it cannot replace an experienced advisor.

This book became a reality through the efforts of a writing team of experienced advisors. For the first edition, two advisors from each of the four regional Associations were appointed as contributing editors and worked both collectively and independently for eight months to complete the project. The advisors and their respective institutions were:

Jane Diehl Crawford	Cornell University	NEAAHP
William Hussey	Brooklyn College	NEAAHP
Zelda Lipman	University of Miami	SAAHP
Norman Sansing	University of Georgia	SAAHP
Julian Frankenberg	University of Illinois	CAAHP
James Nielsen	Western Illinois University	CAAHP
Cynthia Lewis	San Diego State University	WAAHP
Ronald McCune	Idaho State University	WAAHP

For the third edition, the following advisors were added as contributors:

Carol Baffi-Dugan	Tufts University	NEAAHP
Debra Kirchhof-Glazier	Juniata College	NEAAHP
Sally Olexia	Kalamazoo College	CAAHP
Anthony Smulders	Loyola Marymount University	WAAHP

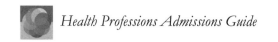

Peter Van Houten, Health Professions Advisor at the University of California, Berkeley and member of the Editorial Review Board to the NAAHP, contributed the chapter on "The Minority Group Student" for the fourth edition. In previous editions, this chapter was written by Harold Bardo, Southern Illinois University College of Medicine.

Each contributing editor brought valuable experience, abilities and insights to the publication. The editors and NAAHP are indebted to them.

For the fourth edition, members of the Editorial Review Board to the NAAHP were asked to review and suggest changes where needed. John Klein, chair of the ERB, coordinated this effort. Members contributing were:

Robert Cannon	University of North Carolina-Greensboro	SAAHP
John Friede	Villanova University	NEAAHP
John Klein (chair)	John Carroll University	CAAHP
Lee Ann Michelson	Harvard University	NEAAHP
Alice Sima	Benedictine University	CAAHP
Marliss Strange	University of Oregon	WAAHP
Peter Van Houten	University of California, Berkeley	WAAHP

For the fifth edition, the following advisors were added as contributors:

Paul Crosby	University of Kansas	CAAHP
Cecilia Fox	Occidental College	WAAHP
Helen Pigage	United States Air Force Academy	WAAHP
Edward Trachtenberg	Clark University	NEAAHP

For the sixth:

Laurence Savett	Macalaster College	CAAHP

For the seventh:

Glenn Cummings	Princeton University	NEAAHP
Karen deOlivares	Southern Methodist University	SAAHP

Finally, for this edition, the following advisors were added as contributors:

Kirsten Peterson	Allegheny College	NEAAHP
Consuelo Lopez Springfield	University of Wisconsin, Madison	CAAHP

We also must acknowledge the assistance of the staff from the national office of NAAHP. As always, Kristen Cota, Media Specialist, was critical to producing this publication. Appreciation is extended to the NAAHP Advisory Council members - those individuals affiliated with the respective professional school associations who reviewed earlier manuscripts for usefulness and accuracy. The associations are:

American Association of Colleges of Nursing	American Physical Therapy Association
American Association of Colleges of Osteopathic Medicine	Associate of Accredited Naturopathic Medical Colleges
American Association of Colleges of Pharmacy	Association of American Medical Colleges
American Association of Colleges of Podiatric Medicine	Association of American Veterinary Medical Colleges
American Dental Association	Association of Schools and Colleges of Optometry
American Dental Education Association	Association of Schools of Public Health
American Medical Association	Association of University Programs in Health Administration
American Occupational Therapy Association	Physician Assistant Education Association

Finally, a very special note of thanks to Brice Corder, who brought the original project to fruition and shepherded it through its first four editions.

Carol Baffi-Dugan and Rob Cannon, Editors

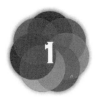

PLANNING FOR YOUR CAREER

INTRODUCTION TO CAREERS IN HEALTH CARE

Health care has been one of the most rapidly expanding areas of our society during the past decade. Careers in this area have expanded, both in numbers and in the variety of opportunities. "As the largest industry in 2006, health care provided 14 million jobs — 13.6 million jobs for wage and salary workers and about 438,000 jobs for self-employed and unpaid family workers. Of the 13.6 million wage and salary jobs, 40 percent were in hospitals; another 21 percent were in nursing and residential care facilities; and 16 percent were in offices of physicians." [1] Students aspiring to a health career hope it will provide an ideal balance in their working lives. They expect their profession to offer intellectual stimulation, economic security, and they wish to take pride in a service that they perform for society. Many careers in health care provide these rewards.

A reassuring aspect of most health care careers is relative stability of employment. Currently, a major effort is being made to encourage students to consider careers as nurse practitioners, physician assistants, and primary care physicians. The U.S. Department of Labor forecasts a high demand in most health care fields. These are also jobs that must be performed where the need exists.

A second characteristic of health careers is that they offer geographic mobility. Any community large enough to support a hospital will require a wide spectrum of health professionals. Aerospace engineers, stock traders or magazine editors all have a limited number of places where they can pursue their careers. By contrast, employment is available for a nurse, physician assistant, medical technologist, or family physician across the country.

However, most health careers offer limited chances to advance (vertical mobility). In general, you are trained to perform a specific function, and that is what you do. A medical technologist runs various tests on body fluids and tissues. Twenty years from now s/he will be doing essentially the same task; only the equipment and tests will have changed. The head of that laboratory will often be a pathologist (M.D. or D.O.), although that is in the midst of change. This lack of vertical mobility occurs at the doctoral level as well. A dentist, for example, has had little chance for "promotion." However, the limited vertical mobility is often offset by advances in the field. Many careers in health care require life-long learning. There is a widening array of areas into which a health care professional can bring his/her expertise. Increasing opportunities for additional education and change of specialties in mid-career exist. These routes often require further training in residency or in other specialized programs.

You will also find that it is rather difficult to change fields within health care. If a nurse wishes to become a physical therapist, s/he must go back to school for several more years, get a new degree and pass a new licensing exam. Generally speaking, when you choose a specific health career you are choosing your life's work. Make sure you have considered your choice carefully.

Another characteristic of the health care field is stratification. The doctoral fields such as medicine, dentistry, optometry, podiatry, veterinary medicine, physical therapy, and pharmacy all take about eight years of schooling, four undergraduate years and three to four more in professional school. You may then spend several years in a residency program. Other health professions generally require bachelor's or master's degrees and take four to seven years to complete. The doctoral level fields have higher average incomes while the bachelor level fields have moderate incomes. Tables I and II at the end of this chapter provide you with representative incomes for both doctoral level generally and other degree programs.

This stratification is perhaps most important in terms of independence and authority. Most of the American health care system still accords more autonomy and authority to physicians and others with doctoral degrees. Health professionals in areas that don't require these advanced degrees are important providers and members of the health care team but in many cases they ultimately respond to the physician's orders. Even those with advanced degrees may have limitations, which vary from state to state. For example, a family physician may write a certain prescription. A pharmacist may be aware of a newer drug. Although s/he may not be allowed to substitute it the pharmacist may consult with the physician and contribute his/her knowledge about the new medication. A physician assistant may have his/her own docket of patients but must technically rely on the supervision of a physician. A physical therapist may have a private practice but may not be legally allowed to treat a patient without an order from a physician. There is definitely greater recognition of the increasing importance of physical therapists, nurse practitioners, physician assistants and other health care providers, however there are still some differences in level of responsibility and independence that you must weigh as you choose the career that is right for you.

There have been many changes in the past twenty years in the delivery of health care. Insurance companies and managed care are playing much larger roles in the management of the health care system. Technology is having a tremendous impact on diagnosis and treatment, as well as the financial and ethical dimensions of health care. And, patients have more direct access to information and have become more informed and often demanding consumers. We encourage you to explore these different dimensions as you make your decision about a career.

CHOOSING A HEALTH CAREER

"Health professions" cover a broad spectrum that includes careers at the doctoral, master, bachelor and associate degree levels. When choosing a career within the field of health care, or deciding whether a health career is appropriate for you, we suggest asking and developing answers to the following questions:

1. How much do I wish to deal with people? Great variety in skills, interests and personal characteristics are needed for various health professions. For many people, such as nurses, pediatricians or occupational therapists, a warm and caring personality is one of the most desirable attributes. Others, such as medical laboratory technologists, pathologists or medical illustrators, have little or no contact with patients. For a surgeon, it may be more important to have good manual dexterity and be calm under pressure than to have an outgoing personality. One of the first questions you should ask is how much you wish to deal directly with people.

2. Am I comfortable studying science? You do not need to be a science "whiz" for all health care areas. Some programs demand much more science study than others, but preparation for all health care careers involves some laboratory science study.

3. Am I prepared to enter an area where I will have to spend time and effort keeping up with developments in my field? Competent practitioners have an obligation to their patients to give the best care available. If you are not willing to continue studying throughout your career you will not be a competent health care provider, thus compromising your malpractice insurance, and/or your license.

4. Am I comfortable in a health care setting? Some students fail to anticipate the effect of spending much of their life in the company of sick, disabled or dying people. With the aging of the American population, much of your work may be geriatric. Many students assume that they will be working in a comfortable, middle-class setting. However, the greatest health care needs are in inner-city neighborhoods and isolated, impoverished rural areas. Do you have a spirit of service? Are you emotionally able to deal with a wide variety of people? You should consider exploring your future career and gaining a better understanding of the discipline by pursuing relevant extracurricular activity.

For example, volunteer your time in a hospital, research laboratory, public health agency or clinical setting. You will gain insights that will permit you to make a more informed decision about the health career you wish to enter. Not all of health care is as glamorous as sometimes portrayed on film and television.

5. Am I a team player? Health care is increasingly a group activity where a successful outcome depends upon each member of a medical team performing his/her specific function.

6. What lifestyle do I envision? Some health care careers include many emergencies and long hours. Different specialties have varying levels of responsibility. Do you wish to deal with life-and-death situations? A career that involves long hours or high stress leaves you less time and energy for family life and leisure activities.

Entering a health care field involves great commitment. You must commit time and often many years to obtain the credentials needed for licensing. You then have a commitment to your patients, which is deeper than the obligation that many other professionals have to their clients. Before committing yourself to a health career, you will be wise to take the time to get a clear picture of the realities of your chosen profession and of your own abilities, needs and aspirations. You can use the chapters of this book that discuss various health professions, as well as the appendices to begin a thorough investigation of various health professions

PLANNING THE PROGRAM OF STUDY

High School: Essential Courses and Related Experiences

High school is an early step along the path to your career. If you have a tentative interest in a health career, you can start to focus on that interest while you are in high school. The advantages are that you can do some reality testing to see (1) whether you like the field and (2) whether you enjoy and can master material in science and math classes that are a prelude to those required in college as preparation for health careers programs. Your exploration in high school, in part, should lay the foundation for college courses.

The educational foundation you establish during these years is important for all that is to come later. Some students decide within the first two years of college that they want to pursue a health career. They then find that they are deficient in foundation courses that others have completed during high school. Students who take inorganic chemistry in college without having had chemistry in high school often find the appropriate introductory course difficult. It is not uncommon for these same students to lack a math background. Physics may be a struggle for those who have not had math at least through trigonometry.

Unquestionably, the high school student anticipating a health career is best advised to enroll in a college preparatory curriculum that includes physical and life sciences, preferably the most advanced courses offered. The following courses are recommended for the high school student: mathematics, through precalculus; at least one year of biology, one year of chemistry and one year of physics. Because written and oral communication are essential for a health practitioner, you will need courses in English.

Although courses will help focus your career interest, work and extracurricular activities will give you a taste of the real world of health care. Work in a drug store; volunteer in a hospital or nursing home; babysit a child with cerebral palsy. Such experiences have helped other students decide on their future careers. Although they may not immediately give you a "yes" or "no" answer, they should help give direction to your further explorations. Some high schools offer a Health Occupations Career class, which can acquaint students with the diversity of health careers.

Advanced Placement (AP) courses can be a two-edged sword. They do offer you the opportunity to explore some challenging material in high school and yet not all health professions schools will accept AP credit alone as fulfilling their prerequisites. You have the option of declining the AP credit and taking the course in college. This can be a difficult decision. You must ask yourself how good the high school course was, and how much you learned and retained. Is your good score on the test really indicative of knowledge? Was the laboratory experience adequate? On the one hand, you do not want to waste time repeating material you already know, but on the other hand, you want to make sure you have a firm foundation on which to build your future knowledge. It is particularly important to discuss this with your advisor; the decision may also be affected by your selection of a major and/or the health professions schools to which you intend to apply. Wherever you attend college, you will want to seek the advice of the health professions advisor before you decide whether to use your AP credit to fulfill health careers program prerequisites. It is the responsibility of these advisors to assist students in academic and career planning. These advisors are valuable resources, as much information can be acquired from your health professions advisor, but you must make the decisions.

Choosing an Undergraduate Institution

High school students who are considering a doctoral health professional career wonder what college or university would be best for their undergraduate preparation. You should know that "premed" or "predent" are programs available at most institutions, although most undergraduate institutions do not offer a specific major in these areas. Health professions schools require only a few specific college courses for admission: a year each of general chemistry, general biology, organic chemistry, general physics and English. Any university or college with science departments can offer you preparation for almost any health profession. At most institutions you will not need special permission to take these courses. For example, a "premed" is any student with the dedication, work habits and academic skills needed to complete these rigorous courses.

Sometimes high school students are under the mistaken belief that it will be helpful to attend an undergraduate institution that is associated with a medical school. There are no data that show this to make any significant difference in your chances for admission. Most professional schools like to have a diverse student body, which represents a variety of colleges, majors, ethnic groups, socioeconomic classes, etc. Optimally, they want good students of fine character regardless of their institution.

Some institutions offer "combined degree" programs in which those accepted are assured admission to a professional school from high school. These programs are designed to attract outstanding candidates to those institutions. Students good enough to get accepted to a combined degree program should have little difficulty gaining admission by the normal route (four years of undergraduate study) so long as they maintain high academic standards. Unfortunately, it is a decision that must be made early in one's life. You need to weigh the merits of assured admission against your educational and personal goals.

The most important factor in selecting an undergraduate institution for preprofessional studies is how comfortable you feel in that environment. No program or institution will "get you into professional school." You must get yourself in. Yes, a good advisor can help. But you must do all those labs, you must take the tests, write the papers and get good grades. You must take the admission exam and travel to your interviews. Much of your effort as you try to gain admission to a doctoral profession will consist of sitting in a room with a science textbook and working on the problems at the end of each chapter. That room may be in Boise or Boston, San Diego or South Bend. What will be important are your efforts and your abilities.

BACCALAUREATE-LEVEL ACADEMIC REQUIREMENTS

The Doctoral or Diagnostic Fields

There are health professions whose practitioners are entitled to use the title "Doctor" and whose responsibilities includes diagnosing as well as treating a problem. All involve four years of professional training usually following a bachelor's degree. After completing this lengthy and arduous training, you are entrusted with the highest level of responsibility for your patients. In return, society offers you prestige and substantial financial rewards associated with the profession, and the privilege to exercise a great deal of independent judgment in caring for others. (See Chapter 5.)

The undergraduate preparation for the doctoral fields is similar. The following college level courses with laboratory for each science course are required for most doctoral programs: a year each of: Biology, General Chemistry, Organic Chemistry, General Physics, and English. Some dental, optometry and veterinary schools require only one semester of Organic Chemistry. Some schools also require a course in Biochemistry.

Many schools have additional requirements such as mathematics, psychology or advanced biology courses. Most professions publish reference books that contain detailed requirements for all member schools. However, the courses listed here meet the minimum requirements for most doctoral health programs. Much information about professional organizations and specific schools/programs is now available on websites. See the appendices in this book as well as your health professions advisor for specific details.

Credit for Work Done in High School

While many professional schools want to see grades in prerequisite courses, a considerable number will accept credit based on special examinations such as Advanced Placement (AP) if your undergraduate institution grants you credit toward graduation. In chemistry this gives you the dubious privilege of starting directly with organic chemistry. If you receive AP credit for a full year of physics, this will generally suffice. If you receive AP credit for general biology courses, however, most professional schools want you to continue and take a year of advanced biology with laboratory while in college.

Choice of Major

No particular undergraduate major is required for admission to health professions schools. In general, your chances of admission will not be affected by your choice of major. While biological sciences is the most common health professions major, representing about 47% of those in professional schools, the acceptance rate of biology majors is slightly lower than average. This does not mean that a Biology degree is less desirable; simply that a larger proportion of the applicant pool chose to major in this academic discipline. Students majoring in humanities and social sciences constitute only about 12% of medical school applicants, but their rate of acceptance is generally higher than average, because students majoring in these fields represent a smaller part of the applicant pool. The acceptance rate for students majoring in physical sciences is also high. Those who major in the allied health professions generally have a more difficult time competing. Choose your major based on what you want to study, although if your goal is to become a physician, it may not be helpful to earn an allied health degree first because admission committees often prefer a broad but rigorous liberal education.

The abilities to read, write, and think critically and to do well in science are vitally important for successful admission to health professions schools.

Since you have a wide choice of subjects in which to major, your decision should be based on an honest assessment of your interests and talents. You may also want to choose a major or add a minor that offers an alternate career path if you change your mind about a health career or are unable to gain admission. You are strongly urged to view your undergraduate years as a time for intellectual growth, not solely as a means to an end. Professional schools want students who have proven themselves not only in the required science courses, but also in the humanities and social sciences. They will be looking to see if you allowed yourself sufficient depth and breadth in your studies. The ideal candidate shows not only academic competence, but also evidence of strong, independent judgment and motivation for lifelong learning.

Getting Started

Make sure you are thoroughly familiar with the information provided by your health professions advisor. At some institutions your health professions advisor will be your only academic advisor. In others, especially universities, a faculty member in your major department or advising center serves as your primary advisor. You should obtain whatever written material is produced by the health advisor, visit the website, and/or attend information sessions arranged for health professions students. Whatever advising system is in place in your institution, be sure to familiarize yourself with it and take advantage of it. Freshman year is spent taking general college requirements and getting started in the required science courses. Your first goal should be to set up a schedule that meets these requirements and with which you are comfortable. There should be balance between the laboratory sciences and humanities. You should not overload yourself with "killer" courses, or seek out easy classes in an effort to inflate your credentials. You do want to establish a firm foundation on which to build your academic record. The major you choose will also be a factor in course selection; some majors have sequenced courses that must be taken prior to moving to advanced courses in that discipline. Make sure you speak with your health professions advisor when making up your class schedule. Be frank about your strengths, weaknesses and goals. Your advisor will help make sure you meet both college and professional school requirements. But in the final analysis, it is you who will have to decide each semester what is best for you. It is your academic record that will determine your attractiveness as a candidate for admissions to professional school. Keep in mind that admission committees seek students who have attained educational breadth along with meaningful community/public service.

The Middle Years

The bulk of the first three years of college will be spent taking general college requirements, getting started on your major, and completing those courses required for professional school. A significant goal during this period is to maintain a good academic record.

You need to realize that an academically poor semester or year does not necessarily mean the end of aspirations for admission to a health professions program. At some time during your college years, personal, family, financial or health problems may affect your studies. These barriers are not insurmountable if you prove you can handle your problems and if your subsequent record is good. Of course, one strong semester will not counteract several years of mediocre work. However, professional school admissions committees will respond positively to a steady upward trend in your academic record and hope that you will continue to improve even more during your professional studies.

You are also encouraged to get involved in some extracurricular activities to increase your enjoyment of college and to become a well-rounded individual. While experience working in a hospital or other health or research setting may not be required specifically, it is generally agreed that professional schools value such experiences and look for them. Consider also the importance of providing a service to one's community. These experiences can serve to solidify your career choice and to let the admissions committees know that you are familiar with the field. You must convince the admissions committees that you know what you are choosing and are sincerely motivated to serve others.

It is to your advantage to maintain regular contact with your health professions advisor during these years. S/he can assist you in creating your schedule, offering advice if you get into academic difficulty, helping you find research or summer program opportunities, and generally serving as a "sounding board." When you apply to professional school, your advisor may be asked to submit a letter of evaluation, which will be more valuable if s/he gets to know you well. It is a good idea to prepare a personal profile that you can give to those writing letters. Consider preparing an autobiographical sketch that provides information about your accomplishments and goals.

The undergraduate experience should be enjoyable, a time for intellectual growth, and an opportunity to experience new ideas and make lifelong friends. When you are studying almost every waking hour in professional school, or working eighty hours a week during residency, you will look back fondly on those college years.

Two-Year and Four-Year Institutions

It makes little difference to most health professions schools whether you begin your education at a two or four-year college or university as long as your work at the four-year school meets the standards for acceptance to professional school. Many two-year colleges provide an excellent education, and a quality applicant will stand out regardless of the institution.

However, there are some problems to avoid if you attend a two-year college. First, make sure you obtain proper advice. If there is no knowledgeable health professions advisor on campus, visit a nearby four-year institution that does have one. Most likely, the health professions advisor will be helpful.

Secondly, there may be problems associated with transfer to a four-year college. Be certain your courses transfer between institutions and avoid trying to transfer a partially completed sequence (e.g., physics or general chemistry), especially if it is taken in a term (semester vs. quarter or vice versa) different than the four-year school.

Finally, letters of recommendation may be difficult to obtain without proper planning. Determine that faculty at the two-year college remember you well enough to write an informed letter. Since letters may be needed after just one year at the four-year college or university, you should begin obtaining letters from faculty and/or the health professions advisor immediately upon matriculation. Check with the four-year college to see if they employ a "committee letter" format and how one pursues this recommendation process.

POSTBACCALAUREATE EDUCATION

More people today who are making career change decisions are deciding to pursue health careers subsequent to earning their bachelor's degree. To prepare for careers in medicine, dentistry, veterinary medicine, or other health fields, it is necessary to complete prerequisite courses, take standardized tests, and acquire health-related experiences. Postbaccalaureate (postbac) programs are designed to meet the needs of a variety of non-traditional students who may be interested in a health career.

Some postbac programs are designed to provide only the basic prerequisite courses. Others may allow students to take upper level courses to improve their GPA. In some postbac programs students take courses along side traditional undergraduate students, while in others, students take courses designed solely for postbac students. Most postbac programs can be completed in two years or less.

Admissions requirements and costs for postbac programs vary considerably, and completion of a postbac program in no way guarantees admission into medical, dental, or other health profession schools. Information about postbac programs can be obtained from colleges and universities that offer them, on the NAAHP website (www.NAAHP.org/resources_postbac.htm).

TABLE I
REPRESENTATIVE INCOME
IN THE HEALTH PROFESSIONS*

Doctoral level — minimum of 8 years of postsecondary education

Professional Title	Number in the Profession	Median Annual Income
Physicians and Surgeons	227,000	$132 – 259,948
Surgery – General		$228,839
Osteopathic Physician**	52,827	
Dentists	161,000	$136,960
Orthodontist	9,200	$185,340
Podiatric Physician	12,000	$108,220
Optometrist	33,000	$91,040

* Salaries vary widely according to geographic area and particular work situation. Data are from a variety of sources including professional organizations and the 2008-2009 edition of the Occupational Outlook Handbook prepared by the US Bureau of Labor Statistics.

** Osteopathic physicians make comparable salaries to allopathic physicians depending upon whether they are doing primary care or are in a particular specialty. Statistics on the osteopathic profession can be found on the Association of American Osteopathic Physicians website aacom.org. See specifically the "Annual Statistical Report on Osteopathic Medicine."

TABLE II
REPRESENTATIVE INCOME
IN THE HEALTH PROFESSIONS*

Bachelor's, Master's Degree or Clinical Doctorate

Professional Title	Number in the Profession	Median Annual Income
Medical Lab Technologist	167,000	$ 49,700
Nurse (R.N.)	2,505,000	$57,280
Occupational Therapist	99,000	$60,470
Pharmacist	243,000	$94,520
Physical Therapist	173,000	$66,200
Physician Assistant	66,000	$74,980
Respiratory Therapist	102,000	$47,420

* Data are taken from the Occupational Outlook Handbook (see Table I).

1. Bureau of Labor Statistics, U.S. Department of Labor, *Career Guide to Industries, 2008-09 Edition*, Health Care, on the internet at www.bls.gov/oco/cg/cgs035.htm (visited *January 25, 2009*).

APPLYING TO PROFESSIONAL SCHOOL

In the preceding chapter, we encouraged you to think about your people skills, desire to study science, and the importance of staying informed. As you prepare your application to professional school, choose the schools to apply to, and present yourself in your interviews, you should consider developing thoughtful answers to the following basic questions:

1. **What draws me to my chosen career in health care?**

2. **Am I making an informed career choice?**

   - How much do I know about what it is like to be a patient?
   - How much do I know about what it's *really* like to practice the health profession I have chosen.

3. **Do I have a good head?**

   - Do I have the intellectual capacity not only to do the work required by the professional school?
   - Do I have the ability to perform the work required of the professional?
   - Am I open to new ideas? Creative? Have I developed the ability to look at a problem in more than one way?

4. **Do I have a good heart?**

   - Do I understand the meaning of empathy? Altruism?
   - Do I appreciate the importance of the relationship between the professional and the patient ("the doctor-patient relationship")?
   - Am I comfortable with people who are different from me?

5. **Am I prepared to make a serious commitment?**

   - Am I willing to spend the time required to prepare for the practice of the profession and for the practice itself?
   - Am I willing to spend sufficient time with each of my patients to meet his or her needs?

Considering these questions helps you to validate for yourself and for the professional school admissions committee that your career choice is a wise one.[1] You have a number of opportunities to address these questions in the application process: personal essays, supplemental question forms from individual schools, and your interview.

Remember your resume is a summary; you are more than the list of your accomplishments — grades, scores, activities and jobs. The purpose of the application process is to show the professional school admissions committee who you *really* are, and that goes beyond simply recounting what you have done. Beyond your grades, scores and activities, the committee looks for evidence of intellectual depth and personal reflection. You demonstrate those qualities when you thoughtfully describe what you have learned from each of your important experiences. Individual stories help to illustrate the points you wish to make.

Considering the questions outlined above will also help you determine when to apply. Recognize also that:

- The best time to apply is when your application is the strongest. If there are major gaps in your knowledge and/or preparation, you should consider delaying your application until those gaps are filled. Your advisor can help you identify those gaps.
- Since health professional schools often issue acceptances on a rolling basis, sooner is better than later in applying and completing your application.
- While important, it's not all about grades and test scores. Professional schools are looking for human qualities — service to individuals and to the community, for example, and some sort of leadership experience. A good predictor of future altruism is past altruism.
- Professional schools want their applicants to have a sampling of the professional experience, so that they are familiar with the career. Your advisor can help you make those connections.
- Professional schools look for excellence in any major, not just a major in a scientific discipline.
- Professional schools look for scholarship beyond the classroom: research in any subject or other activities that evidence intellectual inquisitiveness.
- Professional schools are looking for cultural competence — a sensitivity and awareness of diversity.

The most important first question is not, "How do I get in?" but rather, "What's the right career for me?" That means making an informed choice. In the pages that follow we expand on the questions raised above and other issues related to becoming a successful candidate to a health professions school.

<u>What draws me to my chosen career in health care</u>? Nearly every serious candidate for admission has the desire to help and to serve. Yet each person has made a unique personal journey. Every story is influenced by different experiences, role models and the communities to which a person belongs. Think about your goals in the context of the variety of health careers (and careers in the helping professions). Doing so can help you answer then whether the career you intend is right for you.

<u>Am I making an informed career choice</u>? A career in medicine, for example, requires at least 7 years after college (4 years of medical school and 3 or more years of residency), a large financial outlay, and commitment to life-long learning. Unless you have some awareness of what being a physician is like, then you are making an uninformed choice. One can gain knowledge about health care professions and the patients professionals serve from:

- Personal or family experience with illness
- Paid or volunteer activity serving others in a clinical setting. You can learn a lot while you deliver flowers to a room, find magazines or other reading material or direct visitors. Be observant and sensitive to others around you. Jot down questions and ask when the people you are working for or with have an opportunity to answer.
- Reflecting on your experience. A favorite question in counseling and teaching, and in interviewing students for professional school, is: "What did you learn from this?" Ask yourself this question often. Ask also, "What did this experience mean to me?" It helps to keep a journal, a record of your reflections.

<u>Do I have a good head</u>? If all that professional schools required was a good academic record, then they could fill their classes with students who have 4.0 grade point averages (GPAs) and perfect admission exam scores. But schools look for more. Consider GPAs and test scores as only a threshold, and an early way of screening for intellectual capacity. One advisor put it this way: "Your 'numbers' may get you into the game. Everything else keeps you in the game."[2] The "intellectual capacity to do the work of the professional" does not require genius, but you should have some aptitude for science, an open mind and intellectual curiosity. These latter qualities enable an individual to explore alternatives in order to look at complex and difficult problems in new and creative ways. The really good professional examines all the information, draws a conclusion, then takes a step back to ask, "Is there yet another way to look at this?"

A career as a health care professional requires a commitment to life-long learning — from teachers and colleagues; from texts, journals and continuing education courses; and from patients. Begin developing the disposition early. When you take a class make an effort to extend your reading beyond that required for class. Look for articles in academic journals that build on concepts taught in class. Look up legislation related to health care, and find out about what is being proposed in your state. Attend special lectures offered at your university or in your community. Look for ones on a variety of topics.

The ability to look at an issue in depth also is an important consideration, often illustrated by undergraduate work in some concentrated area or the extended study of an issue or problem. For example, if you are interested in how patients react to physical surroundings you might take courses in architecture, engineering, psychology and/or anthropology. If you are interested in decisions that are made about when patients are taken off life support, you might take classes in philosophy, public policy and/or political science.

Being a non-science major is not a disadvantage in the application process. Any major is acceptable, as long as science grades are strong, pre-requisites are met, and an applicant has sufficient depth to manage the curriculum s/he will be expected to master.

<u>Do I have a good heart</u>? A career in a health care profession requires more than technical skill. Professional schools carefully look for human qualities in their candidates for admission. A career in health care is built on relationships: between professional and patient, among professionals in the same career, and across professions. Draw upon your experiences and reflections. Reflect especially on the meaning of "the doctor-patient relationship." Look up definitions for empathy and altruism.

<u>Am I willing to make a serious commitment</u>? Be certain that you are aware of all matters related to time, especially the importance of providing adequate time in the individual transaction between the professional and the patient. Commitment is also about the time spent in preparation. Included in this book are resources (on the web and in print) that can help you better understand the type of commitment you will be expected to make to prepare for entering a profession, as well as what you might expect when you do enter that profession. Use the following timetable as a guideline to help you shape your adventure as a pre-health student.

TIMETABLE FOR DOCTORAL PROGRAMS

Many applicants underestimate the time required to complete the application process. You will need to complete primary and often supplementary application material, take admissions tests, submit results of those tests to the professional schools, request evaluation letters, submit those letters to the professional schools and arrange for transcripts to be sent to the schools or centralized service.

An application that arrives just before a deadline may have a lower chance of favorable action. A late application may be viewed as an indication that you may not be truly committed to the career or the school. An application prepared hurriedly in order to meet a deadline may not present you in the best possible way. Finally, an application submitted at the deadline may arrive after many acceptances have already been issued. By the time your file is complete and you have been interviewed, only a few positions may be left in the entering class since many schools use rolling admissions. Everything must be done in a logical sequence and in a timely fashion.

Timetables vary. The following timeline applies to those students who plan to matriculate into health professions schools directly after earning the bachelor's degree.

Freshman, Sophomore, Junior Years
- Speak with a health care professions advisor.
- Take the required courses for admission to a health professions school at a reasonable pace.
- Get some experience related to your anticipated career. Many schools now want to see evidence that you have had some clinical exposure.

Junior Year (Spring Semester/Quarter)
- Speak with a health professions advisor.
- Take the standardized admission test.
- Attend the meeting on the application process, if your school has one.
- Obtain the application.
- Obtain a transcript at the end of the year for your own use in preparation of the application.
- Request that official transcripts be mailed to the individual schools or the application service.
- Arrange for letters of evaluation.

Summer after Junior Year
- Complete your application.
- If you are applying through an Early Decision Program, check to see that your letters of evaluation have been submitted and prepare for interviews.
- Check deadlines for mailing, as they vary for different application services.

Senior Year (Fall Semester/Quarter)
- Complete supplemental (secondary) applications.
- Arrange for letters of evaluation to be mailed.
- Interviews are arranged at the discretion of the professional school.
- Send an updated transcript at the end of the fall semester/quarter if a school has asked for it. In most cases, this is a good idea even if schools do not request it.
- Begin preparation for financial aid. (See the "Financial Planning" section of this guide.)

Senior Year (Spring Semester/Winter and Spring Quarter)
- Interviewing may continue.
- Submit financial aid applications.
- Decision time
- Speak with your health professions advisor.
- Choose a school.
- Make alternative plans.

Late Summer and Early Fall after Senior Year
- Begin professional school.

Unless you decide, in consultation with your health professions advisor, that you should delay applying until you can establish a more viable candidacy, complete the application process on schedule, even if your test scores are not competitive. If you decide to repeat the admissions test in the summer or fall, check the box on the application indicating that you plan to repeat it. This notifies the professional program to delay final action on your application until receipt of your new scores.

Normally, professional schools will notify you of your status after the admission committee has acted on your application. You can expect to fall into one of four categories: acceptance, rejection, being placed on an alternate or wait list, or being placed on hold. The last category merely means that the committee considered your application but did not make a final decision. You are less likely to be notified of this status than of the other three.

After receiving an acceptance, you may request a deferral for such reasons as study abroad, doing research or other personal reasons. Some health professions schools will grant a one-year delay in matriculation, if it is sufficiently justified.

NON-TRADITIONAL STUDENTS

More and more students enter the application cycle later than the above timetable because of a change in majors, a change in interest or a change in careers. Some non-traditional students have a bachelor's degree in a non-science field without the required science and math courses. In fact, there are increasing numbers of people who decide to enter a health professions program later in life (from age 25 to over 40). They have been referred to as non-traditional students, and their numbers are increasing.

Many colleges and universities offer a complete year of inorganic chemistry, organic chemistry, biology or physics during a summer session. This can allow a student to take the admission test in August and begin the application process at that time. It is inadvisable to commit yourself to so compact a schedule without consulting with an advisor and determining if you are able to produce a record that will make you viable for favorable consideration.

Many colleges offer postbaccalaureate programs with a compressed schedule of science and math courses. (See Chapter 1.)

Students who are citizens of other countries may have a significantly reduced chance of obtaining admission to health professions schools unless they can finance their entire education. Many schools have both a citizenship and residency requirement. However, there are some private and a few public schools that will accept foreign citizens. These students should contact their health professions advising office for the names of the professional schools that will consider their applications. Resident aliens, those with a green card, are generally treated like U.S. citizens.

STANDARDIZED TESTS FOR ADMISSION TO PROFESSIONAL SCHOOL; METHODS OF REVIEW; REVIEW COURSES

Essentially all health professions doctoral programs require a standardized, nationally administered test, specific to the profession, to support the application for admission. Why is there a reliance on standardized tests when evaluating a student for admission? First, grades alone do not tell the complete story when predicting whether or not an applicant has the aptitude and intellectual capacity to complete a very demanding professional program in the health sciences. Further, an applicant may have attended an undergraduate institution whose academic standards are not particularly well known to the admissions committee. The standardized exam helps establish the validity of the student's grades.

For example, the Medical College Admission Test (MCAT) is a computer-based test offered many times throughout the year (www.aamc.org/mcat). Other tests like the Pharmacy College Admission Test (PCAT) are offered only at specific times. Information about which test may be required can be found on the official websites of the professional organizations (see Appendix D). The following provides information applicable to preparing for standardized admissions tests in general

- Test Format and Content. One of the first things a student anticipating taking such a test should do is to learn as much as possible about the test, both its content and format. Knowing how you will be tested is an important part of preparation. One should plan to utilize the official practice examinations available from publishers of the test as well as their handbooks that provide information about the examination and how it is scored. Practice tests can be important in identifying areas of weakness and strength and in allowing the student to become more familiar with the format of the test and the level of difficulty of questions. Practice tests should be taken under conditions approximating real test conditions, particularly regarding the time available for the test. Most health professions admission tests will have a reading comprehension or verbal reasoning section. Some also require essays.

- <u>Review</u>. The greatest value of a careful review may be the feeling of confidence you develop as you become increasingly familiar with the material to be tested. An organized, systematic review of the topics to be tested is important. For biology, chemistry, physics and other achievement tests, planning the program of study should include taking the required subjects before these tests are taken.

  Some undergraduate colleges and universities offer an in-house review of science topics (general chemistry, organic chemistry, biology, and physics), and several have prepared review books with problems often supplemented with commercially available study guides and practice tests.

  Some students take a commercial review course before taking these admission tests. The greatest disadvantage in taking commercial review courses is that they are expensive, usually costing $1700 or more. Some commercial review courses offer a reduced rate for students on significant financial aid, if they provide documentation from their health professions advisor and/or from the school's financial aid office. Especially for students with poor test-taking skills and those with less self-discipline to review on their own, the cost of a commercial review course may be worth the price, in order to get considerable experience with practice problems and thereby sharpen their test-taking ability.

- <u>Study Groups</u>. Some students form study groups to prepare for the exam.. Others prefer to review on their own, using commercially available materials to supplement their class notes and textbooks.

- <u>Timing</u>. Whatever method is chosen to review the material for the test, it is best to begin well before the test date. A specific block of study time should be set aside. This review schedule should then be followed faithfully. It is much better to study on a daily basis rather than attempt to review huge blocks of material during a short time. Your class notes, tests and textbooks are particularly valuable resources. The emphasis ought to be on familiarizing yourself with concepts learned previously rather than on learning new material. The questions are often posed so that application of general principles is stressed much more than regurgitation of facts. You must know the facts, but you must also be able to apply these facts in solving problems.

  Professional schools vary regarding the acceptable interval between the time the test was taken and matriculation. Plan to take the test so that your scores will be valid within the acceptable interval.

There are no tricks or strategies that can substitute for knowledge of subject matter, particularly in the science sections. Try to get a good night's sleep before the test and arrive at the test center in plenty of time before the test. Eat well before and during any breaks. And, easier said than done, try to remain calm before entering the testing room. When you actually sit down to take the test or when taking a practice test under simulated conditions, certain tactics may help avoid errors and improve your score.

- Pace yourself. A timer is visible on the testing monitor. Do not spend a great deal of time on a difficult problem or question, only to not answer the easier ones for lack of time. All questions count the same.
- Read through the entire question carefully and be certain that you understand the point being tested before responding. A choice among the early answers may appear correct until you read further and find a better answer. There will be sufficient time for most people to read all questions carefully, unless they are slow readers.
- Do not waste time with questions that will require involved calculations or otherwise use a great deal of time, even if you feel that you could eventually get the right answer. As time begins to run out, make sure you leave sufficient time to provide an answer.

- For the writing sample, the best preparation is to practice writing. One useful technique is to get in the writing habit by keeping a daily journal. You should try sample essay questions from previous exams.

In order to enable your health professions advisor to better counsel you on where to apply, check the box on the registration or test form that will release your test scores to the advisor. This information also helps in the preparation of summary reports, but individual scores are never released without written authorization from the student.

If your scores are not as good as you had anticipated, you may need to repeat the test. However, this decision should not be made hastily. Ask yourself the following questions:

- Are my scores consistent with my grades? If not, why not?
- Did I prepare adequately and conscientiously for the test?
- Will I have the time and the motivation to prepare properly for a second test? Merely taking a test over is no guarantee that your scores will improve; scores may go down as well as up.

Your best source of information and advice when considering whether or not to repeat is usually your health professions advisor.

If you believe you are a poor standardized test taker, address the problem early. In some cases this is due to poor reading skills. Some students score poorly on admission tests because of learning disabilities. If this is the reason for poor scores, federal legislation guarantees you certain rights if you have had a professional evaluation that establishes that you have a learning disability. Depending upon the diagnosis, this may include granting additional time for the test because of reading difficulties, or it may allow a person who is easily distracted by noises or movement to be isolated during the test. If you believe that your low scores on an admission test are caused by a learning disability, discuss this possibility with a knowledgeable advisor. It is expensive to take tests that diagnose the condition and allow it to be certified, but keep in mind that some of our most distinguished health professionals suffered from such problems. If you have the motivation and the academic aptitude to become a health care professional, there is little reason to abandon this dream because of dyslexia or some comparable disability.

APPLYING

Choosing the schools to which you want to apply

As you consider different schools and choosing among those in different locations ask yourself: these questions:

- What sort of city do I want to be in for the next four years — big or small?
- Is it important for me to be near people who are my "support system" — family and friends?
- If I have a strong ethnic or religious identity, is there a community for me at the school and/or in the city where it's located?
- What's the "culture" of the medical school? Are the faculty members and my peers committed to my success? Does the medical school recognize the importance of the human side of medicine? Of community service?
- What about financial considerations? Is there a state institution that provides financial benefits to its resident students?

Your advisor, and friends and alumni who are currently at the schools you are considering, can help you address these questions. You may be tempted to use rankings, often found in commercial publications. Be wary of this approach.

Rankings are often based on vague or criteria or self-perpetuating ones (such as asking medical school deans what schools they believe are the best.) This could direct you towards schools that are not the best match for you.

Application forms and services

There are two ways to apply to health professions schools: through a centralized application service or through direct application to individual schools. The number of schools using a centralized application service is large and growing so that there are now only a handful that require individual applications. You can find out which schools use a centralized service and which don't by talking with your advisor and by consulting resources listed in Appendix D.

As your application process proceeds and time elapses, check frequently with the application service by phone or online to be certain that material has been received, processed and forwarded to the desired professional schools. Check your email frequently for messages from the application service and specific schools. Disable any filters that may interfere with your receiving those messages.

Centralized Application Services: The centralized application services provide standardized information to each of their participating health professions schools from a single form that you complete. The advantage of applying through a centralized service is that initially only one set of application materials and official transcripts need be submitted, regardless of the number of schools to which you apply. The application services provide detailed admission information to health professions schools and to undergraduate health professions advisors, in addition to processing the primary application.

Appendix B lists the services that oversee the centralized application processes of each professional school association. Most now offer web-based applications. You can access those applications, along with instructions, at the association's website. While advisors no longer receive paper applications from most services, they may have additional material or experience that can aid students when completing the application. Each professional school has its own specific deadline for receipt of the application.

All application services require a basic processing fee, plus a sliding scale fee depending on the number of schools to which you request the application be sent. Certain fee reductions or waivers are available to students with financial need. Check with the respective application service regarding the earliest submission date. Directions about how to complete an application and information on fees are available on the websites for the application services. Read these first rather than calling with questions for which answers are readily available. This enables the people at the application services to handle issues that require clarification and/or special problems that may arise.

Direct application: Some professional schools do not participate in these centralized application services. You must write to these schools individually to request their application materials.

Advanced standing and transfer applicants should also contact all schools directly for application instructions.

Official transcripts are required before or after submission of the application, depending on the health profession. It is important that you know when transcripts are needed and plan accordingly. Application services — and often professional schools — will perform an item-by-item check comparing all courses in the academic record section of your application against your official transcript, and so you should review your transcript prior to submitting it to check for errors. The GPA that they calculate may be lower than that on your transcript since any grade of A+ is changed to an A. The application is copied after grades are verified and sent to all the schools you designate. If you decide to apply to additional schools before the application deadline, you need to submit an additional designation form with the appropriate fees, and your application will be forwarded to those schools.

Make certain that you review all application forms early in the application cycle, so that you understand exactly what is expected of you and so that you give yourself sufficient time to prepare an application that allows you to make the best impression.

Generally, each application requires basic biographical information followed by questions relating to your academic strengths and weaknesses, extracurricular activities, honors, and other matters.

Make certain that you carefully read and follow all instructions. See your health professions advisor, or call the application service or health professions schools, to answer any questions you may have. When you have completed the forms and have checked carefully for errors, submit your materials to the application service, which then verifies and reproduces your application and forwards it to each school you have designated. If there is an application service, individual member schools may then send you supplementary application materials ("secondaries") to complete after assessing your initial set of credentials. Some schools require an additional application fee.

Be sure to retain copies of all materials that you submit as part of the application process. It is also a good idea to retain draft material, since information that you leave out of your personal statement may be worthy of inclusion in response to questions on the secondary application (see below). Submit your application early, since most professional schools have a rolling acceptance system; that is, the admissions committee acts on the application once it is complete in all its parts, including secondaries, letters of recommendation, and interview.

Send academic grade reports, as they become available during the year of application, to all schools where an application is pending. Most schools require only a copy of these transcripts; an official copy may be required after acceptance but before matriculation.

Personal Statement or Essay

Most application forms require a one-page essay; some give a general prompt and others allow even wider latitude in selecting a topic. For many students, this is the most difficult and challenging part of the application process. *Your personal statement should be personal.* There is no universal formula; it may touch on various matters: your personal journey toward your chosen career; important experiences and what you learned from them; the special strengths you feel you offer the profession; your goals for your education and career; how you will contribute to the diversity of your class.

Personal anecdotes are often more effective than pure descriptive passages. A well-written, heartwarming passage about delivering meals to an elderly home-bound person may communicate more about you as a person than a statement simply listing such qualities as compassion, empathy, understanding, and a sense of humor.

If you have anything in your background that you feel needs to be explained, include it in your personal statement. If you missed a year because of illness or family problems, or had a difficult semester because your work schedule was too heavy, discuss it here. On the other hand, do not feel compelled to discuss the only "C" you got, as this will just call attention to it. Make any explanation as positive as possible, stressing what you have learned from the experience. Take responsibility for your actions; excuses create a negative impression. Don't exaggerate. Don't compromise your credibility. Could it be that you are a stronger candidate because you have been through this experience? Ask yourself, as many interviewers will ask, "How did it affect me? How did I grow from this experience?"

Obtain critical feedback about your essay from people whose judgment you trust. Ask a peer and/or an advisor to review your application, particularly those parts that require essays or other extensive text, before you submit it. It never hurts to get another opinion. You may choose to purchase a copy of *Write for Success* (see page 168).

When you are interviewed, the interviewer likely will have read your personal statement and your responses on the supplemental application material. Thus, anything you choose to write about should also be something that you feel comfortable discussing. Make sure you save a copy of your application, including your essay. You should read it over again prior to an interview.

Supplemental application material ("Secondaries")

Upon receipt of the applicant's materials from the centralized application service, each professional school will notify the applicant directly regarding the need for any additional material. Generally, you will be asked to answer a variety of essay questions, some of which may be specific to that school, call for your opinion, or ask you to deal with a controversial topic. Some supplementary applications also request more information about your personal or academic history. Some will inquire about why you are interested in that particular school.

Motivated students quickly complete and submit the secondary applications.

LETTERS OF EVALUATION (RECOMMENDATIONS);
choosing whom to ask

Whether you have the intellectual capacity to do the work of your profession will become clear to the admissions committee when they receive your undergraduate transcript and the scores from your national standardized test. However, there are other qualities upon which you will be judged, such as motivation, maturity, perseverance, judgment, compassion, integrity, interpersonal and communication skills, cultural sensitivity, and the potential for continuing intellectual and professional growth.

Lack of one or more of these qualities is most often responsible for keeping a student with high grades from being accepted; if these qualities were not important, then the incoming class could be selected entirely by a computer. Although some of these characteristics can be gleaned from your application and your interview, evaluation letters are one of the most important sources for describing and appraising these traits.

You can expect that, after initial screening, admission committees will require letters of evaluation. The more personalized and specific the evaluation is, the more valuable it can be for you. Regardless of the system your school uses for collecting these letters, you should understand that it is to your benefit to get to know well a few faculty members, in order to fulfill this requirement when the time comes to apply to professional schools.

There are three general methods used in preparation of a faculty evaluation.

1) The first method uses individual letters prepared by faculty members and others who know the applicant well, with the letters going directly to each professional school to which the student applies.
2) A second method uses a composite evaluation prepared completely by a health professions committee.
3) The third method uses a composite evaluation generally prepared in a health professions advising office. This method uses letters of evaluation from faculty members chosen by the applicant, with summary comments and ratings prepared by the chief health professions advisor.

If your school has a committee system and you cannot use it — you might have transferred into the school and do not know enough professors to contribute to your file, or are a non-traditional student who took much of your work with faculty who are no longer at the school, or prefer not to use it for some other reason — then you may arrange for individual letters to be sent. In such cases, it is a good idea to let your health professions advising office know about it, so that the advisor can assure professional schools that you are applying with his/her knowledge and are not trying to circumvent your school's system. On the other hand, if your school has a committee system and denies you a supportive committee letter because you do not meet their criteria, it is still your prerogative and right to arrange for individual letters to be sent to the professional schools of your choice. Professional schools will accept letters from faculty and make the definitive decision whether or not you qualify to attend their school.

In gathering your faculty evaluations, the most important factor is that your evaluator knows you well and is not just going to submit a standard letter for all his/her A students, another for B+ students, etc. Here are some guidelines.

- Don't be reluctant to ask those whom you choose, "Can you write a strong letter on my behalf?" If the person can't, find someone else.
- If letter-writers are college professors, be certain that they go beyond your grade to describe you as a person.
- Stress the importance of a prompt letter. Give your evaluators both a deadline and sufficient lead time. A tardy letter can hold up an invitation for an interview and/or overall consideration of your application. Keep track of your evaluations; do not assume that they have been sent because the professor said s/he would do so soon.
- Be prepared to furnish your evaluator with additional information about yourself. Let your evaluators know the type of health profession school to which you are applying. Prepare an autobiographical sketch for your letter writers, and make an appointment to discuss your career plans. Tell them why you are motivated to pursue a particular career.
- Professional schools are interested in your science capability and usually require at least two evaluations from science faculty.
- Diversify your evaluations by submitting them from several different disciplines, including humanities and social science faculty.
- If you request an evaluation from a professor with whom you are currently taking a course, suggest that he or she draft the evaluation after the course has been completed. Alternatively, you may want to alert the professor that you will ask for a letter at some future date.
- Faculty with whom you are involved in research or other individual or small-group curricular projects may be in a better position to evaluate you than those who know you as but one face in a large class.
- Letters from physicians, family friends, peers, clergy, etc. come under the category of "character references" and should not be confused with faculty evaluations. If such references are required by some schools, they are usually sent directly to those schools by the persons writing them. Some schools designate the types of letters they prefer. It is usually best to avoid soliciting a letter from political figures, if it is written simply as a favor to a constituent, rather than as an endorsement based on personal knowledge or interaction. Letters from former employers are often of value since they can address such personality characteristics as maturity, responsibility, independent judgment, and interpersonal skills. If you have assisted in any research, especially at a health professions school, a letter from that project director can discuss both your cognitive and personal attributes in a way meaningful to an admission committee. If you have done volunteer work with a health practitioner or in a health care facility, a letter from your supervisor might also be appropriate.

Under the provisions of the Family Educational Rights and Privacy Act of 1974, known as the Buckley Amendment, you have the right of access to all educational records including letters of evaluation sent to health professions schools by your health professions advisor and/or your faculty. You can either waive or retain your right to read these letters. Admission committees often prefer confidential letters because they assume that a more candid and, therefore, a more helpful evaluation will usually be written if the professor knows that the confidentiality of the evaluation is to be respected. Be assured that your letters are confidential and will only be sent to the institutions that you designate. That said, it is your civil right to insist on the right of access to your academic records and evaluations.

THE INTERVIEW

When a letter arrives inviting you to an interview, you have every reason to be exhilarated since most schools only interview a fraction of their applicants. Your application and transcripts have been carefully scrutinized, and the reviewers have deemed you to be an acceptable candidate for strong consideration. Read the instructions that come with the invitation to the interview very carefully and respond promptly. Delaying your response or unnecessarily putting off the interview may imply lack of interest in the school. You may choose to use a written resource to help you prepare for your interview. [3]

See the interview as reciprocal. The medical school representative is, of course, interviewing you, but you are also interviewing the school. The interview is an opportunity for you to enhance and complete the picture of who you are, to show that you can think and speak clearly, and to illustrate how you form a relationship. At the same time, the medical school is trying to recruit really good candidates, and so you want to use the time to address any questions you have about the school. Not only is the interview your single most important opportunity to express or explain yourself to the admission committee, it is also your opportunity to learn something about the institution firsthand. It provides you the opportunity to ask questions about its programs and faculty and to tour the facilities. You can gain information that might not be available in the institution's website, literature, and other public documents.

Most health professions schools use an interview to assess a number of personal qualities deemed necessary for successful academic progress and professional practice. Regard the interview as an opportunity to present yourself as one with realistic goals and aspirations. It helps to decide in advance what it is that you want your interviewers to know about you and your special strengths. Some career counseling centers at undergraduate institutions provide an opportunity for a mock interview and videotape the student for a later debriefing of strengths and weaknesses during the interview.

The interview provides the admission committee, through its representatives, with the opportunity to meet you, verify your credentials and supplement its knowledge of you. The interview is also used to obtain explanations and insight into any problems encountered with your application. For example, you may wish to explain health or family problems that adversely affected your academic performance.

Some professional schools offer you a choice of an on-site interview or a regional interview closer to your home or school. Regional interview are usually conducted by alumni, often in their office. An advantage of the regional interview is its lower cost in time and money. However, the on-site interview gives you an opportunity to view the facilities and the area around the school and to interact with students. If you are already traveling to a particular city or region for interviews and have not yet heard from other schools nearby, it is quite proper to contact those schools. If they had planned to grant you an interview, they may be willing to arrange it at that same time. For air travel, special rates may be available through a discount ticket program.

At the interview, most schools use a one-to-one format, with one or more interviewers. A few schools use a committee interview, with three or four persons on the panel. Interviewers are typically clinical faculty, basic science faculty, or students, especially where multiple interviews are the custom. These personal interviews are relatively unstructured and usually last from thirty minutes to an hour.

Interviewers will likely evaluate you to assess your personal qualities, including:

- Your understanding of the career: Do you know what it's *really* like and what patients need from you as a professional?
- Your motivation: How strong is your desire for your chosen career? The interviewer might want to further test your motivation by posing questions regarding your experiences in the field you have chosen.
- Your level of maturity and judgment: How well and logically do you think on your feet? Are you emotionally stable and mature?

- Your intellectual curiosity: What is the evidence that you recognize the importance of life-long learning? How well do you learn from experience?
- Your interpersonal skills: Do you communicate with the interviewer easily and clearly? How well do you relate to the interviewer? What's the evidence that you can work well with others? Since you will be caring for patients with both physical and psychosocial problems, the interviewer will be interested in assessing your ability to relate to, communicate with, and empathize with people from various cultural and ethnic backgrounds.

Interview Tips

Preparation for your interview involves thinking about your goals, strengths, weaknesses, and the information you most wish to communicate to the admission committee. This preparation is of enormous help if your interviewer begins the session by saying, "Tell me about yourself." Think about the current state of the profession and how you stand on various issues related to the profession. There are no "correct" answers for these questions; the interviewer wants to determine whether you have thought seriously about the profession and can defend your positions in an articulate manner.

- In advance, learn about the school by looking at its website, reading their publications and by talking to students on that campus before your interview session. A common interview question is "Why are you interested in attending our school?"
- If possible, arrange to arrive at the school early enough to avoid stress and to look around and get a feeling for the campus.
- Spend time with current students and find out more about the school and its atmosphere. Are the faculty and your fellow students committed to your success? Does the school attend as much to the human side of medicine as the technical part? Some schools help you make arrangements to stay overnight with a student or at inexpensive accommodations. Your health professions advising office may give you names, phone numbers and addresses of alumni from your college who are current students there.
- The school will inform you in advance where you are to report for the first interview, general information session, or tour. Often you will be told the names and positions or titles of the interviewer(s). The interview can be "open- or closed-file." For the latter, the interviewer has not been given your letters of evaluation or information about your academic background. But even in closed-file interviews, your personal statement and your answers to questions on the secondary are often available.
- Refrain from anything that might be viewed as objectionable by the interviewer, such as gum-chewing and nervous mannerisms. Maintain good eye contact. Display your best "professional manner." Dress professionally, but comfortably, and remember that this is not the time to make a statement with your clothes, hairstyle, jewelry, perfume or deodorant. While it is impossible to eliminate all the stress inherent in the interview process, the most important thing to remember is to conduct yourself naturally and calmly. First impressions are important.
- Try not to appear defensive. If you make an error in one of your statements and realize it, admit it. Never try to bluff a response. Try to be open-minded and willing to learn. Understand the difference between questions requiring factual responses and those asking for opinions. Do not be reluctant to take the time to think before responding; a complex question requires some thought. Videotapes of mock interviews show that the silent interval is usually shorter than you imagine.
- Do not be reluctant to express your feelings during the interview. Be open about your concerns. Many interviewers ask that you continue if you are too brief; be prepared to give more detailed explanations. They often ask about your family and the kind of relationship you have with family members. The open-ended format gives you an opportunity to describe accomplishments while giving background information. Don't sound boastful, yet take the opportunity to make the committee aware of positive factors about you that would be difficult to present in any other way.
- If you feel that the interview went badly, many admissions officers will respond favorably to a request for second interview with a different interviewer.

Some schools give you a comment sheet after the interview that asks for feedback. It is important and appropriate to express your concerns as soon as possible, especially if the interview went badly. Such comments are normally considered confidential by the administrator in charge of the interview process. Your health professions advisor can usually help you decide how to handle this situation, and you should certainly inform her/him of any problems you encountered, particularly with regard to what you believe to be illegal or improper questions.

Many applicants write or email thank you notes to their interviewer after the interview.

You may choose to purchase a copy of *Interviewing for Health Professions Schools* (see page 168).

TWO PLUS TWO DEGREE PROGRAMS

Many allied health and B.S. nursing programs are said to be "two-plus-two" degree programs. This term refers to the fact that high school graduates enroll in the college or university of their choice for two years of study as a "pre-nursing" or "pre-med tech" student. In these two years you would complete requirements for admission to the professional program, then apply for admission to the professional school early in the spring semester of your sophomore year. If accepted, you would begin two years of professional study the following fall, your junior year in college.

NON-ACCEPTANCE

Some students are not accepted on the first try. Here are a few possible reasons.

- There are more qualified candidates than places in the first year class.
- The application process reveals too many gaps in your preparation for professional school.
- Grades and admission test scores may be inadequate. Ask yourself, "Have I done my best?" Don't make the mistake of interpreting a rejection from the professional school as one based solely on your test scores. There may be other reasons. The best way to find out is to ask.
- There is inadequate or unclear evidence of motivation and altruism. The best indicator of future altruism is past altruism. Ask yourself, "What's this all about? Do I *really* want this career?"

For help in addressing the reasons for non-acceptance, get advice about remedies from an admissions officer at two or three of the schools that rejected you and from a health care professions advisor.

If you are really motivated, don't give up. Re-apply when your application is stronger. Many have been accepted on the second and third try. Many regard the interim time as especially productive and fulfilling.

There's more about non-acceptance in a subsequent section of this manual.

AND FINALLY...

Recognize that applying is a complex process. If you have emotional ups and downs during the process, be assured that others have had the same experiences and have been successful. While more than 42,000 applicants apply for about 19,000 first year places in U.S. allopathic medical schools, for example, your chances of acceptance are far greater than 1 in 2 if you are a strong applicant.

Use your advisors. Whether you are a current student or an alumnus or alumna, if you haven't already done so, make an appointment soon to talk to your advisor in depth about this process, and don't be reluctant to speak with the advisor more than once.

References

1   To complement your experiences in making an informed choice, here are some good resources, all of which are in paperback:
- Laurence A. Savett, M.D. *The Human Side of Medicine: Learning What It's Like to be a Patient and What It's Like to be a Physician*, (Westport, Conn.: Greenwood Publishing Group, 2002).
- Rachel Naomi Remen, M.D. *Kitchen Table Wisdom.* (New York: Riverhead Books, 1996); and My Grandfather's Blessings. Stories of Strength, Refuge, and Belonging. (New York: Riverhead Books, 2000).
- Kate Scannell, M.D. *Death of the Good Doctor*, (San Francisco: Cleis Press Inc., 1999).

In addition, there is a lengthy bibliography of health-related books on the NAAHP website at www.naahp.org

2   This observation and others have been gleaned from the wisdom of health professions advisors and medical school admissions officers at regional and national meetings of the National Association of Advisors for the Health Professions.

3   *Interviewing for Health Professions Schools*, www.naahp.org/publications

AFTER THE APPLICATION

Once your application has been submitted, events will dictate the concerns you will have from that time forward. While you will be involved in interviews, you can also turn your attention to what happens after the admissions committees make their decisions. If you are accepted, one of your first concerns will be to develop a plan for meeting the financial demands of attending a health professions school. On the other hand, if you are not accepted by any school, you will need to be concerned with "What happens now?" This chapter seeks to provide you with some guidance for responding to each of these possible outcomes.

FINANCIAL PLANNING & AID

Including tuition and living expenses, the total cost of attending a four-year health profession program can exceed $250,000. Costs of programs vary widely, depending in part on the type of program, its length, and whether or not your tuition is partially subsidized by state taxpayers. Some of you may be fortunate enough to have sizable family assets with which to pay for part or all of your education and training. Most are not so fortunate. As a consequence, it is important to begin financial planning for your health professions education even as you begin your undergraduate program.

The Association of American Medical Colleges has developed a program called FIRST (Financial Information, Resources, Services and Tools) that offers valuable information for college students planning to become physicians, and much of the information is also helpful for students planning to enter other health professions. It can be found online at www.aamc.org/programs/first/start.htm.

Minimizing Undergraduate Debt

Try to hold to a minimum any debt you might assume while completing your undergraduate studies. Interest which compounds over the time necessary to complete the undergraduate degree and the health professions program will add substantially to your overall debt load at the completion of your program. Do not carry a balance on credit cards, and do not tempt yourself with a larger credit line or more credit cards than you can use responsibly. Debts during college can make it more difficult, even impossible, to finance a professional school program. It is also vital that you maintain a clean credit record. This cannot be over stressed. If you have any reason to believe you have a poor credit history, you should request a copy of your credit report. If there are negatives on the report, you must make every effort to resolve these problems.

Where do you go for specific information about financial support? You should first exhaust all scholarship possibilities at your undergraduate school. This can be handled by a Scholarship or Dean's Office, or a Financial Aid Office. Need-based support is usually handled by a Financial Aid Office. Most financial aid available through that office will be in the form of the College Work Study Program (CWSP) and a variety of grant and loan programs. The CWSP should be used to the greatest extent possible before tapping into loan programs. Most loan programs have a maximum total amount that can be borrowed, and some of these serve both undergraduate and professional programs, so it is to your advantage to carry as much of this eligibility over to your professional program as possible.

Learn to distinguish between needs and wants. Make a budget and stick with it! You will thank yourself many times over in the future when you begin repaying loans that have been accumulating since your undergraduate years. Strategic planning for your overall financial needs for both undergraduate and professional education, with the help of your undergraduate college or university Financial Aid Office, will pay you many dividends. Working part-time is fine as long as it does not undermine your academic performance. Your first priority is academic success and developing competitive credentials for admission to health professions schools.

You must also be concerned with the cost of the application process. For example, the cost of applying to and interviewing at ten professional schools (a reasonable number) might come to $3,500 or more, including the standardized examination fee, a centralized application service fee, supplemental application fees and travel for interviews. Don't let this cost limit your application horizons. Even though this expense may seem formidable, it is actually a small fraction of your total cost of attending a health professions school. You should look upon this cost (as well as the cost of your professional education) as an investment in your future, or an investment in you as a professional. If you amortize this cost over your lifetime, it actually is a small price to pay to achieve the desired goal. If you plan for this cost, you can avoid using credit cards.

Financing a Professional Education

Even though the cost of health professions education has risen dramatically in recent years, financial support is usually available to complete even the most costly program. In general, you will find that major financial aid will have to come from a variety of loan programs. Most students enrolled in graduate health profession programs receive some form of financial aid. There are two main types of funds available to these students. The first type comes from a series of different loan programs, including the federal Stafford loans and private loans designed specifically for health profession students. To access these funds, you must be a U.S. citizen or have a Permanent Resident Visa. The second type of funds is usually referred to as institutional or need-based financial aid. These funds include both loans and scholarships. They come from several sources — the professional school, the federal government, and private foundations — and are distributed by the Financial Aid Office at the school you attend. As these funds are limited in amount, most professional schools must ration them and may use an analysis of parental financial resources (potential parental contribution) to determine the student's eligibility.

The financial aid application process begins between January and April prior to the professional school academic year, when you submit detailed information about income and assets on the Free Application for Federal Student Aid (FAFSA) form and indicate all schools to receive your federal financial aid data. From this information will come a determination of financial need, which the Financial Aid Office will use to develop your financial assistance plan. If you apply for need-based aid, your parents' income information is sometimes part of this analysis. It is absolutely essential that you and your parents keep good financial records (complete tax returns early during the year you will apply for financial aid) for this process to be completed efficiently.

The health professions school Financial Aid Office is required to calculate a Cost of Attendance figure for each academic year. Under ordinary circumstances, the amount of financial aid you receive from all sources, including merit and service obligation scholarships, cannot exceed this figure. Federal financial aid regulations specify what types of expenses can and can not be included in the cost of attendance. Among the allowable costs are tuition, fees, books, educational supplies, and living expenses. Costs that are not allowed include car payments, prior consumer debt, and moving expenses. Once again, from a financial perspective, the best way to start professional school is free of consumer debt.

Loans

The following is a listing of some of the major and most often used loan programs you may wish to research. These programs are constantly being revised and funding limits change. Seek up-to-date information from each school's Financial Aid Office. Even the availability of some programs may be in doubt in any given year, so ask about any individual program. As mentioned earlier, eligibility for an aggregate total sum of money from several of the programs may extend across undergraduate and professional educational years. That is, borrowing less money as an undergraduate will increase the number of dollars available to borrow when you are in the health professions program. These loans generally offer the lowest interest rates available:

1. Federal Perkins Loan: A subsidized program for students with exceptional financial need.
2. Federal Subsidized Stafford Student Loan: For students with financial need.
3. Federal Unsubsidized Stafford Loan: Not need-based, but interest is not subsidized.
4. Federal Loans for Disadvantaged Students (LDS): Need-based loans for students from disadvantaged backgrounds.
5. Graduate PLUS Loan: Federally guaranteed, low interest loans for graduate and professional students.
6. Private Alternative Loan Programs. Generally, these programs allow students to borrow the difference between their cost of attendance and the other financial aid they have received. These funds are provided by banks, and the loans are not guaranteed by the federal government.

Medical school students may be eligible for the Primary Care Loan (PCL) program. This provides funds for those students who commit to going into a primary care residency and practice (primary care includes Family Medicine, General Pediatrics, Internal Medicine and Preventive Medicine). This program is a need-based loan and thus requires the submission of parental information.

Other special loan programs may be available, depending on the health professions school where you enroll. An excellent source of information on loans, budgeting, credit, and debt management is provided by the AAMC FIRST (Financial Information, Resources, Services, and Tools), found online at: www.aamc.org/programs/first/start.htm

Loan Consolidation Programs

To fund your education, you may need to borrow from several different sources, and to simplify repayment, you may want to consider consolidating your student loans. Most federal loans are eligible for consolidation into either a Federal Family Education Loan (FFEL) or Direct Consolidation Loan. Although loan consolidation may simplify repayment, it may not be financially advantageous, and, therefore, must be investigated carefully before being undertaken.

Similar loan programs are available from the federal government for other health professions schools. For example, DENTALoans is a suite of federal loans specifically designed for dental students.

Service Obligation Programs

If you plan to go to allopathic or osteopathic medical school, dental or optometry school, or other health professions school, a major source of support can be the United States Armed Forces Health Professions Scholarship Program, which includes separate programs for the Air Force, Army and Navy. These programs pay all tuition and fees, buy required books, materials and supplies, and pay a taxable stipend for rent and other living expenses. In return, you will be obligated to serve as a health professional on active duty (holding the rank of captain or equivalent) one year for each year of support with a minimum requirement of three years. You may be required to spend 45 days on active duty each summer if your professional school program schedule allows it. When possible, postgraduate medical education (i.e., internship and/or residency) must be done in a military program. Time spent in postgraduate medical education is not considered "payback time." It does, however, count toward military retirement and promotions. These scholarships are competitive and are awarded to the most highly qualified students. Your health professions advisor should be consulted to help you develop the best strategy for consideration for such a program. You need to consider carefully whether you wish to pursue this avenue of financial support. It would normally be a big relief to have your medical education expenses covered. You need to decide if the limits on where and how you practice, and the required payback time, are acceptable in exchange for their support.

A limited number of National Health Service Corps Scholarships are available for individuals planning primary care careers. Payback occurs in the form of practicing in an under-served location. Details of this program are similar to the Armed Forces Program with a two year minimum commitment. Selections are made from enrolled first year medical students.

Scholarships

A wide variety of scholarships is available through federal and state government programs, through private businesses, organizations, and individuals, and through professional schools. Eligibility criteria also vary widely, but may include academic merit, financial need, underrepresented minority status, or intention to serve in an underserved community.

Working with Financial Aid Offices

The precise details of financial aid programs change from year to year. Help in sorting through these programs is available through the Financial Aid Office at the health professions school. These offices view it as their responsibility to help you meet your financial aid needs with the best possible mix of money from personal sources, scholarships and loan programs.

Finally, everyone involved in this process agrees that financial planning is an absolute necessity. As you move through your undergraduate program and on to a health professions program, you will appreciate that fact many times over. In all cases, you should seek the opportunity to speak with an institution's Financial Aid Office. It is ultimately your responsibility to learn about all of your financial aid options, and successfully manage your debts.

IF YOU ARE NOT ACCEPTED

Your worst fears may be realized when you receive that last thin letter. By now you know the lines all too well. "We are sorry to inform you that we are unable to offer you a place in the class entering in the fall." Although it is true, it does not help much that the letter goes on to state that the school regrets that the large number of highly qualified applicants makes it impossible for all of them to be accepted and they hope that you will have an opportunity at another school. You may know you are qualified, and that you would be successful, if given the chance. The choices admissions committees make between qualified candidates can seem arbitrary, and sometimes unfair. And, you may not receive your last letter until late in your final academic year, or even after you have graduated.

If you are typical of most applicants who are not accepted, you may feel rejected, angry, embarrassed, sad, or depressed. For some of you, it is nothing more than a temporary career crisis. You have acknowledged the possibility that this could happen and have planned accordingly. You at least have some sense of direction at this point and have considered the options that are open to you. For others, it is not only a career crisis, but also an identity crisis. Although this may not bring much comfort, you should know that many do not succeed on their first try. The question is, "What do I do now?"

Now What?

Just as you sought advice on your initial applications, you now need advice with which to plot your best course of action. Some of you will not seek help at this point because your mind is closed to anything other than immediate reapplication. This may not be realistic, so begin to gather facts about what you will need to do. One source is your health professions advisor, although your feeling may be that you do not want to go near his/her office at this point. However, your advisor is more objective than you can be and has experience helping many applicants deal with this situation. Should you happen to be near a health professions school, an admissions officer at that school may also give you assistance.

Unfortunately, you are less likely to consult these individuals than you are to talk to family and friends. The advice they give is often less objective than what you will receive elsewhere, and likely focuses on the issue of reapplication to professional schools or what you can and should do to achieve your primary goal. They sympathize with your plight and are concerned for your welfare, but they do not have the up-to-date information, experience, or perspective to advise you best. There is nothing wrong in talking over your situation with family and friends, but you are cautioned not to base your decisions solely upon their advice.

You need to conduct an honest appraisal of yourself as an applicant, which may mean re-evaluating what you have done to date. You need to know if your credentials were not competitive enough, and, in order to answer that question, you also need to know why others were competitive enough for admission. It is not at all difficult to find out the accepted applicants' academic profile. Your health professions advisor may have such information readily available. If not, one of the professional schools to which you applied can tell you about their average grades and test scores or even give you national averages. Did you apply to enough schools? If yes, did you include schools that afforded the best probability for admission? Did you consider state of residency? Was your application timely? These questions and many more need to be answered.

Reapplication

Now that you have had time to reflect, and have sought preliminary advice about your lack of success, you may decide to seriously pursue reapplying. Persistence can pay off and the statistics for reapplicants are promising enough to justify serious consideration of trying again. If so, it is time to adopt a positive approach. Rather than focusing on why you were not accepted, you need to focus on how you can become more competitive. Why reapply if you do nothing to improve your application?

You may be able to enhance your qualifications for admission by performing well in additional courses, or, if necessary, by re-taking some courses. Is it possible to take enough courses in one year to raise your GPA significantly? It is hoped that you did not compound the problem by letting your grades slide in your senior year because you anticipated admission on the first try. If you do need to raise your GPA, should you consider pursuing another major field of study, or should you pursue graduate work in biology, or another area? The answer to these questions is, "It depends." If you select either option, you should consider the other prospects that a second degree or graduate program can lead to, beyond just accumulating hours and getting grades. In other words, your plans should focus on what you will be able to do with that degree if you are once again unsuccessful with your application. Will it lead to an alternative career that, although perhaps not as satisfying as your first choice, would be a realistic and acceptable option for you?

It is possible that you are a "late bloomer." Perhaps you had a rough start in the early undergraduate years because the adjustment from high school to college was difficult. Or perhaps you had not decided to pursue a health career at that time and lacked the motivation to perform well academically. In any case, you should know that all is not lost. Health professions admissions committees are interested in an accurate assessment of your potential for academic success and will, therefore, consider trends in your grades. Taking additional undergraduate courses or successfully completing a graduate program may help demonstrate a transformation. The idea is to address directly any questions or concerns an admissions committee might have about you as a candidate.

You may be able to develop your qualifications for admission by re-taking the admission test. If you decide to re-take the exam, it will be important to consult with your health professions advisor, and develop a plan for improving your scores. Your strategy should include a thorough review of core science concepts, as additional time will have passed since you took the courses covering this material.

It is true that not all applicants with above average grades and test scores are accepted to professional schools; this demonstrates that health professions schools are looking for more than just academic potential. Again, your health professions advisor will be able to give you more information about your credentials in this regard. Although he or she may not have access to the interview reports from professional schools, your advisor often has established relationships with admission staff members that may improve your chances of getting a response. If they were channeled through his or her office, your advisor should also have access to the letters of evaluation. However, if they were confidential, your advisor will not be able to reveal the contents to you. Remember that professional schools are looking for more than numbers (grades and test scores), and although these additional characteristics are more difficult to assess, an appraisal of your strengths in these areas is necessary.

You may be able to improve your qualifications for admission through gaining additional health care experience, and engaging in significant scientific research, social service, teaching, and/or leadership activities. If all you need is experience, you may want to consider devoting a year to a health related service program. Your activities will, in turn, help you earn strongly supportive evaluation letters, and give you more to present in your applications and interviews.

Once you identify the qualifications you would most like to develop, it would be wise to consult with your health professions advisor, and decide how to accomplish your goals. You may want to develop and implement your own independent improvement program, perhaps by continuing your education at your undergraduate school. Alternatively, you may want to apply for admission to postbaccalaureate (after bachelor's degree) programs designed to help reapplicants become more competitive.

Postbaccalaureate Programs

According to Baffi-Dugan and Lang (1999), there are a wide variety of postbaccalaureate (postbac) health professions programs. One of the biggest distinctions is between programs designed for students who decide to become health professionals after completing education in other areas, and those designed to enhance reapplicant qualifications. Some are designed to help both career changers and reapplicants. In addition, many programs are specifically intended to develop or enhance the qualifications of disadvantaged or underrepresented minority candidates. The Association of American Medical Colleges maintains a fairly comprehensive list of postbac programs at services.aamc.org/postbac, with an emphasis on programs designed for students who decide to become health professionals after completing education in other areas.

Beyond the populations they are designed to serve, postbac programs differ widely in the focus and range of support they offer, and in the affiliation agreements they have with particular professional schools. These affiliation agreements sometimes involve counting coursework in the postbac program toward completion of first-year medical school requirements, guaranteeing interviews or a number of openings for program participants, accelerated admissions cycles, and/or offering conditional admission to postbac students who meet academic and admission test criteria. Programs that are relatively comprehensive and those offering affiliation advantages are also likely to be competitive for admission. As in applying to professional schools, it is important to apply to the postbac programs that can best meet your needs.

In addition to target population, support and affiliation agreements, you may want to consider program length, full-time versus part-time involvement, advisor availability and experience, admission test preparation availability, cost and availability of financial aid, location and potential impact on state residency, and undergraduate versus graduate standing. Some programs help you develop other possibilities by leading to partial or full completion of a master's degree, often in health or biomedical sciences.

Opening Other Doors

If you decide not to reapply, it would still be wise to consult with your health professions advisor. It also might be helpful to meet with a general career counselor for help clarifying your career values and goals. When examining alternative careers, it is important for you to evaluate your earlier motivations and goals for a career in health care. What were the challenges, satisfactions, and rewards you anticipated? Examining your own life goals and talents, and matching these to a career can be hard work, but the effort is worthwhile, especially if it leads you to a fulfilling lifetime career.

Perhaps one of the other health care careers discussed in this book could become a satisfying option. See Appendix A for brief descriptions of a number of these health professions.

Some people, who are initially interested in health careers, are also interested in social, helping professions such as teaching, social work, or clinical or counseling psychology. Some are more interested in scientific research, and enter graduate programs in related areas. And, some move on in other directions.

References

Baffi-Dugan, C., and Lang, G. (1999). A Postbac Primer. *The Advisor*, 19(1): 17-21.

Monetary Decisions for Medical Doctors: www.aamc.org/students/financing/md2.
AAMC FIRST (Financial Information, Resources, Services, and Tools): www.aamc.org/programs/first/start.htm

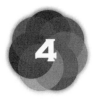

DIVERSITY IN THE HEALTH PROFESSIONS

INTRODUCTION

In our global community, one that is increasingly transnational and mobile, a diverse pool of healthcare professionals is critical in making healthcare available to those needing it most. According to the U.S. Census, nearly half of the U.S. population will consist of racial and ethnic minorities by 2050, about one-fourth of whom will be Latino. Yet, in contrast to the growing diversity of our nation's population, our healthcare industry is not diverse enough. Racial and ethnic minorities comprise 26% of the total population; yet roughly 6% of practicing physicians are Latino, African American and Native American (AMSA). Other healthcare fields reflect similar trends. Coupled with this problem of under-representation is the fact that minority groups have less access to healthcare and receive poorer quality healthcare than today's population at large. Most minority communities are more likely to have family incomes less than 200% of the federal poverty level than whites and less access to culturally sensitive healthcare. Studies have clearly shown that minority physicians are more likely to treat minority and indigent patients and to practice in underserved communities.

Contributing to our nation's growing health disparities is ineffective cultural competency education within the environments of both medical training and patient care. While racial and ethnic diversity contribute to the educational experiences of all health professional students, broadening perspectives and increasing cognitive outcomes for all groups, challenges to building a critical mass of racial and ethnic students remain as Affirmative Action programs are increasingly under assault.

To achieve equity in healthcare, a variety of educational initiatives are nonetheless under way, sponsored by private foundations, professional associations, government, and educational institutions. The Federal Government's Title VII authorizes the health professions education and training programs administered by the Health Resources and Services Administration (HRSA). These programs support the education and training of the full range of all healthcare providers, including physicians, dentists, pharmacists, nurses, psychologists, and public and allied health professionals in education and training through loans, loan guarantees, and scholarships to students, and grants and contracts to academic institutions and nonprofit organizations. Designed to improve the supply, diversity, and distribution of the health care workforce, Title VII diversity programs increase minority representation in the health professions by strengthening the pipeline to a health career. Similarly, the primary care medicine and dentistry programs expand the primary care workforce, while the interdisciplinary, community-based linkage programs facilitate training in rural and urban underserved areas. Together with Title VIII nursing education programs, health professions programs are a critical component of the health care safety net, training a diverse supply of health professionals who are more likely to serve in community health centers and other rural and urban underserved settings.

These organizations realize that to reduce healthcare disparities while promoting compassionate and culturally competent care, diverse healthcare professionals are needed in the educational pipeline. LGBT (lesbian, gay, bisexual, transgendered) people represent a minority of the U.S. population who are also underserved. Expanding the ranks of LGBT practitioners is essential, for all too often, identification invokes stigma and prejudice in healthcare settings. More "out" medical professionals are needed to increase visibility of LGBT health issues in an effort to foster more comfortable and effective treatment of LGBT patients as well as increase awareness throughout the medical community. Sexual orientation is virtually overlooked in population-based national health surveys and among those that do, funding requests for federal support have mostly been denied.

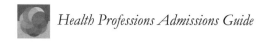

RESOURCES

Building a Support System

Those involved in admissions know that having a support system is a key element in ultimate success. Seek advice routinely from your health professions advisor, as well as other advisors and mentors on your campus. These individuals may be located in academic and advising departments, administrative units, scholarship programs, or multicultural affairs offices. While they may not have comprehensive knowledge of the preparation process for entry into a health profession, they can play a vital role by guiding you toward good resources and helping you clarify your goals. Also, be sure to take advantage of academic support personnel offering assistance through tutorials, learning centers, and academic departments. And do not forget to visit members of the faculty during office hours to discuss your choice of courses and other academic projects. Since you will need faculty letters of recommendation, share your perspectives and understanding of course material with them on a one-to-one basis. Faculty may also be instrumental in helping you to find research opportunities and to explore your academic strengths.

Student organizations offer outstanding opportunities to glean information on health careers, volunteer opportunities, and campus visits. They can help to connect you with others who share your dreams and can support you with study circles. Some may focus on minority or multicultural issues; others may be of general interest. Do not become disconnected! Make sure that you have a healthy cadre of students among whom you may develop leadership skills while learning more about support services.

Websites and Publications

Publications of interest to minority students are often available in your health professions advisor's office. Sections of publications noted elsewhere in this book, and in publications such as *Medical School Admission Requirements (MSAR)* provide valuable information and resources for minority candidates. Another valuable resource is www.aspiringdocs.org. AspiringDocs.org is an initiative of the Association of American Medical Colleges (AAMC) which has been designed to "raise awareness about the need for more diversity in medicine." It is a resource designed to connect you with other students and with the resources you need — everything from summer program opportunities to the latest information on the medical school application process. Osteopathic medical schools have long been committed to promoting diversity in medical school classes. Look for information about osteopathic medicine and the application process on www.aacom.org.

The American Dental Education Association biennially publishes *Opportunities for Minority Students in United States Dental Schools*. Copies of this book are mailed to health professions advisors at colleges and universities. If your college does not have a copy, you can order one. Visit the ADEA website at www.adea.org or call (202) 289-7201. The cost is $10.00. You will find this book has facts, descriptions of clinical specialties, and a listing of special outreach programs. ADEA is now also sponsoring the Explorehealthcareers website, www.explorehealthcareers.org, which offers a wealth of information about various careers, summer internships particularly geared to disadvantaged students, and many other resources. This is a comprehensive and easy-to-use site.

The NAAHP website, at www.naaahp.org, has a section on diversity which offers information on a wide range of health professions and their efforts in this arena. Websites and publications for the different health professional organizations frequently list persons who coordinate minority recruitment programs. These officials are good sources of information and support. They frequently sponsor open houses or advising sessions at their schools or on college campuses that you should attend. Contact them to be placed on mailing lists to receive up-to-date information and guidance, as well as feedback on the progress of your preparation or status of your application.

Keepsake is an annual publication directed to minority students that contains interesting articles, listings of programs, and inspiring stories. It is delivered free to college admission offices. Check the "Resources" section at the end of this chapter, as well as the Appendices in this book for a more complete list of publications and websites. Many of them have specific sections geared toward minority students.

Resources for Enrichment and Research

A valuable source of guidance and support may be found in a wide variety of enrichment programs located either on your campus or at various health professional schools. At some colleges, there are programs to introduce minority and/or disadvantaged students to recruitment, research and clinical opportunities. These programs offer many advantages to those who participate by providing guidance and support plus the important opportunity to test your interests and capabilities for a career in that field. As all health professional schools desire to see evidence of firm and clear motivation to serve in the field, these opportunities to explore your intended field should be pursued eagerly.

In addition, a number of summer enhancement programs are offered to minority/disadvantaged students by health professions schools. Visit aspiringdocs.org (the interactive website created by the AAMC), www.explorehealthcareers.org, as well as www.naahp.org/resourcesminopp.htm for lists of various programs. These summer programs include varying combinations of research, clinical experiences, entrance test preparation, academic review, and study skills development. Since they are held at the health professions schools, participation can provide you with a good understanding of the life of students and practitioners in those health professions. Those who take part often return to their campuses with renewed focus, enhanced skill, and a better understanding of what lies ahead in their pursuit of a career in a health profession. Ask your health professions advisor or minority contact person at health professional schools for details on these programs and for information on applications. Some of the publications and websites mentioned in this book provide listings of such programs. Among them is the Summer Medical and Dental Education Programs (SMDEP), a free, six-week academic enrichment program for freshmen and sophomores with activities including science and mathematics, career development, clinical experiences, financial planning and study skills seminars. It is important to remember that applications for some summer programs are due as early as December, with many other deadlines in January and February. Recommendation letters and essays are often needed for these programs, so plan ahead to meet application requirements.

Postbaccalaureate Programs

A number of people decide that they want to enter a health profession late in their college careers, or take a detour in their science coursework. For that reason many schools offer programs that are called "Postbaccalaureate" ("postbac" for short), through which students can complete the courses they lack for entrance into a health professions school after they have earned their bachelor's degrees.

Other postbac programs may offer opportunities for students who have already taken all their prehealth required science courses to improve their academic records by taking additional courses and thus become more academically competitive for admission. A few postbac programs are intended for minority students, but most are open to all students. If a postbac program interests you, discuss your options with an advisor. Most often, those hoping to improve their academic records need to show strength in science courses. Carefully assess your potential and motivation to significantly improve your grades. As with every step in the preparation process, thoughtful self-assessment and appropriate responses will increase the chances for success. Consult with those experienced in minority admissions matters to gain additional insight into ways to enhance your application. Frequently, applicants do not take the appropriate steps to improve their credentials. If the science grade point average needs improvement, only additional course work in the natural sciences is appropriate; more volunteer work or a job will not help when you need to remedy a grade deficiency. You need to take the appropriate action to make yourself more competitive.

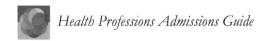

A FEW NOTES ON THE APPLICATION PROCESS

Minority Status

Some application processes offer candidates an opportunity to identify themselves as minorities on the basis of race, ethnicity, and/or disadvantaged status. Moreover, some applications invite applicants to write a short statement on diversity. Make sure you take the time to thoughtfully complete these short essays. Additionally, self-identification may well result in opportunities to provide additional information on your background, including the characteristics of home and community, demonstrated interest in your community, financial status, or other special circumstances. It is important to respond to such questions carefully so that the schools will gain a clear picture of you and any obstacles or special challenges encountered, especially those which you have overcome. This will provide them with insight on how you will respond to the demands of a health professions school. The latter issue is important. School officials want to be sure that all accepted applicants have the drive, determination, and support they need to successfully complete their academic program.

Selecting Schools

School selection is important. The admissions process is subjective and somewhat unpredictable. Yet, with good information, careful thought, and informed advice, you can increase your chances for success. By carefully considering what the schools say and by reading descriptions of the curriculum offered in publications and websites, you can make informed choices.

In most cases, public schools give preference to state residents. Yet, public schools will often accept highly qualified out-of-state under-represented minorities. Private schools normally have no state preferences. If you are applying to medical schools, reading the Medical School Admission Requirements (*MSAR*) and similar publications for other health professional schools, you can increase your chances for a successful application.

Information on minority enrollment in each school is often available. For example, see the *MSAR* or the *ADEA Official Guide to Dental Schools*. However, remember that such figures do not reflect how many minority students were accepted — just how many enrolled. While the number of minority applications has increased, enrollment has not followed suit. Diminishing numbers don't reflect the goal within the influenced by them. Attempt to determine your "fit" at the various schools through pre-application visits, interview trips, and contact with the schools, including members of minority student groups and minority contact officials.

Your advisor can also help. S/he may be able to provide you with information on the profile of applicants who are from under-represented groups on your campus who have been accepted at various health professions schools, or a composite sketch of the "successful applicant." Take this advice into consideration but remember that there are few absolutes in the admissions process. Most advisors recommend applying to a range of schools and not just to "places I dream of attending." A realistic variety of choices, again resulting from a careful self-assessment and review of the schools' admission policies, will be helpful in obtaining success.

Financial Aid

The cost of applying to and attending a health professions school is a concern for all applicants. Be sure to review the financial aid section of this book and to consult references to locate sources of financial aid.

If you have extreme financial limitations, you might be able to receive fee reductions or waivers for required admissions tests and the applications themselves. For medical school applications, information and application materials about the Fee Assistance Program (FAP) are available at www.aamc.org/students/amcas/fap.htm. By receiving an AMCAS fee waiver you not only reduce the cost of the initial application, but also may be able to obtain a waiver of the fee for the secondary application. Be sure to ask for fee waivers early in the process, as time-consuming documentation will likely be required. Also consult minority contact officials at the health professions schools for information on fee waivers, as well as special sources of financial aid for minority students. At some schools it is possible to obtain a fee waiver just by requesting it. Some professional schools also have funds to help competitive applicants defray the costs of traveling to interviews; and some schools have scholarships for minorities, especially highly competitive candidates eager to help underserved populations.

Most schools will automatically consider you for their various scholarships based on your financial aid application. Some schools may require you to send a separate application for each individual scholarship. When applying for the scholarship, check the background of the person whose name the scholarship is set up for and the reason it exists. This will help you with the appropriate tone of your application/essay for the scholarship. Talk with your pre-health advisor and/or the admissions staff at the schools to which you have been invited for interviews for more information.

Since 1946, National Medical Fellowships, Inc. (NMF) has helped to improve the health of low-income and minority communities by increasing the representation of minority physicians, educators, researchers, policymakers, and health care administrators in the U.S. training minority medical students to address the special needs of their communities; and educating the public and policymakers to health problems and needs of the underserved populations. This non-profit organization has awarded more than $39 million to over 28,000 participants, each demonstrating financial need.

Lastly, scholarships for Disadvantaged Students (SDS) are federal need-based scholarships based on exceptional financial need as determined by parents' income and assets, even if the applicant is an independent student. The applicant must come from a disadvantaged background, based upon family income or environment. The amount and the number of awards are based on the allocation of funds from the federal government. Contact individual schools regarding application process. For more information about the scholarships themselves go to bhpr.hrsa.gov/DSA/sds.htm.

See pp. 25-28 in Chapter 3, "After the Application," for more complete information on financing your education.

Some Final Words of Advice

Society at large will be better served when disadvantaged low-income, minority, LGBT, and non-English speaking populations are fully integrated into a diverse pool of health professionals, helping to make healthcare equally accessible to all. It is important for pre-health students to be aware of the people, resources and projects working to diversify the medical community by recruiting, educating, and supporting minorities of various backgrounds. We encourage you to pursue solid information by speaking with advisors, admissions representatives, practitioners, and professional organizations. Seek web information and attend meetings of student organizations that will help you on your journey to self-growth. And use every available opportunity to gain biomedical research and clinical experiences, networking skills and, above all, scholarly attainment in all areas of intellectual pursuit.

SELECTED WEB-BASED SOURCES OF INFORMATION FOR MINORITY/ DISADVANTAGED STUDENTS

www.aspiringdocs.org, a website sponsored by the Association of American Medical Colleges (AAMC).

www.aacom.org, the website for the American Association of Colleges of Osteopathic Medicine.

www.explorehealthcareers.com, a comprehensive website on the health professions including career descriptions, summer listings and articles of interest.

Joint Admission Medical Program (JAMP), www.utsystem.edu/jamp an initiative by the Texas legislature aimed at providing opportunities for highly qualified, economically disadvantaged undergraduate students who want to pursue medical education.

National Network of Latin American Medical Students (NNLMS),www.nnlams.com.
National Medical Fellowships, Inc., 5 Hanover Square, 15th Floor, New York, NY 10004; 212/483-8880; 212/483-8897; info@nmfonline.org; www.nmf-online.org. (a valuable source of financial aid for minority students).

Opportunities for Minority Students in United States Dental Schools, published by the American Dental Education Association, 202/289-7201; www.adea.org.

The Point Foundation is the nation's largest scholarship-granting organization for Lesbian, Gay, Bisexual, and Transgender (LGBT) students of merit. For medical students, Point Foundation offers the Gay and Lesbian Medical Association (GLMA) Point Scholarship and the Decker Scholarship. www.amsa.org/lgbt/scholarships.cfm.

American Medical Student Association, www.amsa.org.

Student National Medical Association (SNMA), 5113 Georgia Avenue, NW, Washington, D.C., 20011; 202/882-2881; www.snma.org.

The Summer Medical and Dental Education Program (SMDEP), www.smdep.org.

SELECTED HEALTH PROFESSIONS

General Description of the Profession

A physician's responsibilities cover a wide range of functions in the maintenance of health and the treatment of disease, including caring for patients with both acute and chronic conditions and promoting preventive approaches involving substantial patient education. These include diagnosing disease, supervising the care of patients, prescribing medications and other treatments, and participating in the improved delivery of health care. Although most physicians provide direct patient care, some concentrate on basic or applied research, become teachers and/or administrators, or combine various elements of these activities.

Among the 820,826 practicing physicians in the United States in 2007, 282,291 were primary care physicians, as defined by practices in family medicine, general practice, general internal medicine, and general pediatrics. Other active M.D.s specialized in obstetrics/gynecology, psychiatry, various medical specialties (e.g., allergy and asthma, cardiology, dermatology, gastroenterology, neurology, and pulmonology), general surgery, various surgical specialties (e.g., colon and rectal surgery, neurosurgery, ophthalmology, orthopedics, otolaryngology, and plastic, thoracic, and urological surgery), support specialties (e.g., anesthesiology, pathology, and radiology), emergency medicine, and other clinical areas.

Physicians practice in a variety of settings, including group practices, health maintenance organizations, outpatient clinics, inpatient hospitals, laboratories, and academic settings, as well as in industry, the military, and government. Medicine offers a broad variety of career options. New opportunities emerge with each advance in medical knowledge and with each development in the organization of medical services. During the course of a typical day, the activities of many physicians include performing two or more of these professional roles and providing professional services in two or more settings. Most physicians are actively engaged in their profession on a full-time basis throughout most of their lives.

Most medical students graduate after four years of medical school ("undergraduate medical education") and enter residency programs of three to eight years for additional training in a specific medical specialty ("graduate medical education" or "GME"). Training in family practice, general internal medicine, and general pediatrics takes three years; general surgery requires five years; and subspecialty training in disciplines such as plastic or neurological surgery may involve another two or three years. Residents are trainees in the clinical facility in which the training program is located; they earn salaries that in 2006-2007 averaged $43,266 for the first year of residency and increased to $52,654 for the sixth year of residency.

Decision to Pursue the Profession

An increasingly diverse mix of individuals is choosing medical careers. For example, the proportion of women in the applicant pool has increased dramatically over the last several decades. Whereas in the 1960s and 1970s, the proportion of women applying to and matriculating at medical schools nationally was relatively small, in 2005-2006, women represented approximately 50 percent of medical school applicants, 49 percent of graduating medical students, and 42 percent of residents and fellows. More specifically, applicants to the 2006 entering class included 19,293 women (49.3%) and 19,815 men (50.7%). First-year matriculants in 2006 included 8,445 women (48.6%) and 8,925 men (51.4%). At many medical schools, the number of female first-year students in 2006 exceeded the number male first-year students.

Students from racial and ethnic groups that are underrepresented in medicine are strongly encouraged to apply. Consistent with the Office of Management and Budget Directive 15, the AAMC has, in recent years, been collecting self-reported race and ethnicity data about applicants and matriculants in such a way that they are able to identify themselves as members of multiple racial and ethnic groups. Comprehensive information about applicants and matriculants from these multiple racial and ethnic groups for the 2002-2008 entering classes can be found on the Association of American Medical Colleges (AAMC) website at: www.aamc.org/data/facts.

As part of a continuing effort to enhance the diversity of medical school classes, the AAMC initiated, in October 2006, the AspiringsDocs.org campaign. The cornerstone of this effort is the AspiringDocs.org website (www.aspiringdocs.org), which is free and features a variety of resources for prospective medical students, including information about career options in medicine, preparing for the Medical College Admissions Test (MCAT), applying to medical school, financing a medical education, and important deadlines in the application and admissions process. In addition to the information on the new website, the campaign also provides a dose of inspiration for potential applicants by highlighting real-life stories of practicing physicians who have overcome a variety of obstacles and barriers on their way to medical school.

Neither age nor marital status is a consideration in the assessment and selection of medical school applicants, and the number of older applicants and matriculants has increased in recent years. In 2006, there were 1,772 applicants whose age at expected matriculation was 32 years or older. Of those, 467 (26.4%) received an acceptance to at least one medical school. Many medical students are married with children.

What is the Unique Role and Responsibility of the Physician?

Medicine is both an art and a science. A physician develops the skills to interact with a patient, obtain a medical history, perform a physical examination, and conduct and interpret diagnostic and laboratory studies. The results of these efforts are synthesized into a comprehensive diagnosis and treatment plan. Since patients' diseases manifest themselves in idiosyncratic ways, the physician must become skilled in the application of science to solve medical problems, often within short time frames and with limitations on the data that can be obtained within the time available.

A physician's first responsibility is to his/her patient. Of necessity, many patient work-ups will require long hours and an unpredictable schedule. There is great satisfaction for the physician in knowing that s/he has taken care of a patient's medical needs. The spouse and family of medical students need to appreciate the long and demanding work schedules required of busy physicians. By the same token, physicians must learn to be considerate of the personal and social needs of their families.

It is also a physician's responsibility to educate his/her patients and promote healthy lifestyles. After all, the origin of the title "doctor" is from the Latin word for "teacher." Practicing physicians speak of the privilege they feel in being permitted to care for patients and to be of service to the community. The care of a patient throughout the lifespan is a particular privilege and requires the utmost from the physician.

What are the Characteristics of Those for whom Medicine is a Good Choice?

The responsibilities of being a physician require maturity, integrity, perseverance, and character of the highest order. Honesty is critical. Being able to recognize your limitations is also essential. Respecting the rights of others, being tolerant of personal belief systems and life experiences different from your own, and respecting the dignity of each person are some of the qualities that the successful physician will embody.

Critical thinking and problem-solving skills are central. A basic background in science is necessary, although it is not necessary to major in a science. It is important to choose a college major you enjoy and to take sufficient advanced course work to develop skills in critical thinking, analysis, and communication.

A love of learning is important. Medicine continues to evolve as new research is completed and new findings are incorporated into everyday medical practice. Physicians learn from every patient as they advance the boundaries of medical knowledge. Medicine is an intellectually challenging field that requires the individual physician to be intellectually curious and to continue to learn virtually throughout his/her lifetime. Reading current journals, attending medical seminars, and/or contributing to the research literature are important activities for physicians. While many specialties require completion of a minimum number of continuing medical education credits annually to maintain professional credentials, a commitment to lifelong learning is an ethical and moral responsibility of all physicians.

Interpersonal skills and empathy are important in a physician. To be successful in medicine, a person must have strong communication skills (both oral and written) and enjoy communicating with others (both giving and receiving information), working in teams to achieve consensus, providing leadership to a group, and maintaining emotional stability, discipline, and a sense of calm in the midst of crisis.

It is important to be able to handle stress and to cope with adversity. During medical school, most students experience a greatly accelerated workload and demands on their stamina and emotional equilibrium. The practice of medicine entails significant demands on the physician's time and involves critical decision-making, often in life-threatening situations. Therefore, individuals considering a medical career are encouraged to develop appropriate stress and time-management skills.

Outlook for the Future

The Bureau of Labor Statistics projects that employment for all physicians and surgeons will grow faster than the average for all other occupations through the year 2014. Discussion continues about the number and type of physicians that will be needed to serve the health needs of the country in the future. Experts studying the physician workforce believe that the United States may experience a deficit of physicians in future decades if the size of medical school classes does not increase or if additional medical schools are not established in the near future, and that population demographics may result in the need for more physicians trained in the medical and surgical specialties. As a result of these projections, the Association of American Medical Colleges recommended in June 2006 that medical school enrollment increase by 30 percent during the next decade. Demand for physician services is expected to continue to rise with the ongoing increase in the population in the United States, especially among those over the age of 65. In addition, one-third of current physicians are over the age of 55 and expected to retire by 2020, and recently graduated physicians are not expected to work the same number of hours per day that prior generations of physicians reportedly worked. You will want to be a well-informed observer about, and perhaps a participant in, these discussions as they progress, as well as about efforts at multiple levels to ensure that adequate health care is available to all citizens and especially to those who are currently medically underserved.

Planning a Program of Study

General Information

There are 130 M.D.-granting institutions in the United States. While there are some individual variations among schools, most require at least two semesters (or three quarters) each of English, general biology, general chemistry, organic chemistry, and physics for admission; the sciences must include relevant laboratories. Although not in the majority, some schools also have a mathematics requirement, and the most frequently mentioned mathematics courses are college math, calculus, statistics, and/or computer science. Although these core sciences are required, no specific major is preferred or required.

All required science courses are typically completed by the end of the junior year of college, the time when application to medical school generally begins in earnest for undergraduate students who seek to enroll in medical school directly after college graduation. Also, these science courses are required for adequate preparation for the MCAT, described in detail in the Introduction. This means that you have only three years of undergraduate study to "prove" yourself if you plan to enter medical school immediately after graduation from college.

Entrance requirements for every medical school in the United States and Canada are listed in *Medical School Admission Requirements* (MSAR), a 400-page guide published each spring by the Association of American Medical Colleges (www.aamc.org/msar). You should become familiar with this excellent resource early in your academic program to determine the specific admission requirements of medical schools in which you are potentially interested. The MSAR may be available in your premedical advisor's office, but it is a good idea to purchase your own copy during the year that you apply to medical school. It is carried by many college bookstores and commercial bookstores, and it can be ordered directly from the AAMC. (See Resources.) Additional information regarding each medical school may be obtained on the AAMC's website at: www.aamc.org/medicalschools.htm.

It is also important to check the policies of medical schools regarding Advanced Placement (AP) and College Level Examination Placement (CLEP) credits. Not all medical schools will accept AP or CLEP units. Generally, if you tested out of one of the basic requirements, a medical school will accept an equivalent amount of credits in more advanced courses in that same discipline. If you have these credits in science or English courses, discuss your academic record with your premedical advisor or with medical school admission officers.

Choice of Undergraduate Major

Since the choice of an undergraduate major is not an issue for medical schools, on what basis should you select an undergraduate course of study? Most premedical advisors and medical school admission officers agree that you should select a major based on your interests and aptitudes, so that you will enjoy your courses and do well in them. Should you change your mind about medicine or not gain admission to medical school, your major might also prepare you for an alternative career choice. Many applicants forget that alternative doctoral-level health careers are available that require the same science coursework and same general academic preparation as that required for medical school, and that these careers can offer the same personal and professional rewards originally sought in medicine.

The Admissions Process

Background

Medical schools seek students who will make good medical students and altruistic, knowledgeable, dutiful, and skillful physicians. They are not inclined to take great risks in selecting members of their classes; they have made a large investment, both economic and social/political, in seeing that the people whom they select for entrance become successful students and practitioners.

Medical school curricula have undergone significant revision during the past two decades as medical schools have made substantial efforts to place greater emphasis on modes of active and clinically relevant learning (e.g., problem-based learning, case-based instruction, small-group discussion) and to reduce passive approaches to medical education (e.g., lecture formats, large-group learning). Substantial investments have also been made to enhance the ways in which students' mastery of content and acquisition of clinical skills are assessed. The use of Objective Structured Clinical Evaluations (OSCEs), simulated and standardized patients, mannequins, and videotaped and computerized clinical scenarios are now standard at many medical schools.

During the first two years of the medical curriculum, students learn scientific material basic to the practice of medicine (i.e., anatomy, biochemistry, physiology, pathology, neuroscience, pharmacology, microbiology, immunology), as well as behavioral science, preventive medicine, medical ethics, human sexuality, and other clinically relevant content. They also master the skills associated with medical interviewing, history-taking, and physical examination. The substantial biomedical science content during these two years results in admission committees being interested in your science GPA, overall course load, and scientific and written communication skills as measured by the MCAT.

During the second two years of the medical curriculum, students participate in required clinical rotations called "clerkships." Each clerkship is typically one to three months in length. Core clinical training usually involves rotations in internal medicine, surgery, obstetrics and gynecology, pediatrics, and psychiatry; many schools also have a required rotation in family medicine or primary care. These core clerkships are supplemented by elective rotations, in which students pursue individual interests and begin the process of identifying their future specialty choice. During the clinical curriculum, students exhibit their personal attributes and personality skills, as well as their abilities in the areas of communication, problem-solving, stress management, and leadership, which will be critical to their success as effective practicing physicians. Suitability for this phase of medical education is assessed by means of information regarding the applicant's extracurricular activities, involvement with others, and communication skills as discussed in letters of recommendation and exhibited in personal essays and interviews with admission committee members.

Factors Evaluated by Admission Committees

Each medical school's entering class is selected by an admissions committee appointed by the dean of the medical school. While the size and composition of the committee varies from school to school, it is usually composed of basic science and physician faculty members and medical school administrators. Many schools also include alumni, local physicians, medical students, and non-medical citizens from the surrounding community. The composition of the committee usually changes somewhat from year to year as some members complete their terms of office and new members are identified.

Admission committee members strive for objectivity in making their decisions. In general, medical schools select for admission those individuals who present evidence of strong intellectual ability, a record of accomplishments, and personal traits indicative of the ability to communicate and relate to patients in a realistic, professional, and compassionate manner. There is emphasis on academic achievement over time, MCAT scores, and multiple personal characteristics and experiential variables, including maturity, judgment, empathy, altruism, persistence, motivation, commitment to service, resilience, and concern for others. Some important determinants of whether or not you will be accepted for admission are:

- academic record
- scores on the MCAT
- content of letters of evaluation and recommendation
- personal statement
- the impression made in your personal interview(s)
- experience in a medical setting, and
- evidence of community involvement and volunteer and extracurricular activities.

Each of these is discussed below.

Academic Record. Your undergraduate record will be a significant factor in predicting admission to medical school. Studies show that the quality of work in subjects taken leading to the baccalaureate degree is a very important predictor of success in basic science classes in medical school. The academic record includes the overall GPA and the science GPA (biology, chemistry, physics and mathematics), as well as performance in each individual course and trends in performance over time. Trends are an important consideration; a poor freshman year followed by improvement during the sophomore and junior years is preferred to a good freshman year followed by a declining record. A good academic record is evidence of high motivation, ability, and persistence — all factors necessary for the successful completion of a medical education.

Grades and academic load are not evaluated in a vacuum, but rather in context of your total time commitments. If during college you worked part-time, played a varsity sport, or otherwise devoted significant time to serious extracurricular activities (journalism, performing arts, community service, student government, etc.), these activities will be taken into account. However, it is necessary for the medical school admission committee to have evidence of your ability to do medical school-level work at an acceptable level. The best way to present this type of evidence is to already have done well during your undergraduate years.

The Medical College Admission Test (MCAT). The Medical College Admission Test (MCAT) is another extremely important factor in evaluating an applicant for medical school. During and after medical school, you will have to pass nationally standardized licensure and certification examinations. Since many of these tests show high correlation with each other, medical schools are most interested in those candidates who have demonstrated content mastery and proficiency in testing by doing well on the MCAT. In addition, studies have shown that MCAT scores are statistically reliable and valid predictors of academic success in the basic medical sciences in medical school. Some medical schools conduct a preliminary screening based entirely on GPA and MCAT scores as a component of the process of selecting those applicants to be interviewed. While it is important to realize that satisfactory GPA and MCAT scores may be necessary for acceptance to medical school, they are not sufficient in themselves; qualitative factors also play a very important role in the admissions process. All applicants, with the possible exception of some students enrolled in baccalaureate-M.D. programs or applying to Early Assurance Programs, must present MCAT scores as a necessary part of the materials supporting their application.

The Letters of Evaluation. Letters of evaluation are discussed in detail in chapter 2. Medical school admission committees generally prefer a composite or committee evaluation to individual letters of evaluation. Many will insist on such an evaluation if you are from a school where a composite or committee evaluation is prepared. Follow the guidelines described earlier, and, by all means, keep in close touch with your health professions advising office in collecting these important supporting documents.

The Interview. Once again, the discussion found in earlier pages can serve as a guideline. At the medical school interview, you should be prepared to answer some rather personal questions about your own background, beliefs, and experiences, as well as questions about moral and ethical issues affecting medicine. Review your record and expect to be asked about your interest in medicine, community and campus activities in which you have participated, and examples of ways you have exhibited leadership, faced up to challenges, and solved difficult problems.

Extracurricular Activities and Work Experience. Medical schools view extracurricular activities as positive signs that you can handle a rigorous curriculum and still participate in campus or community affairs. The level of your participation is more important than the number and diversity of your activities. Commitment, leadership, service, responsibility, and the ability to interact effectively with others are among qualities that medical school admission committees seek in applicants. These activities include community service, campus involvement, participation in research, outside jobs, interests, hobbies, etc. It is a myth, however, that extensive involvement in meaningful extracurricular activities will compensate for a modest academic performance. It may instead indicate to an admissions committee that you have poor judgment, skewed priorities, and/or inadequate time-management skills.

Health-Related Experience. In addition to the service component, an important value of volunteering in a hospital, doctor's office, nursing home, or health clinic is to help clarify the validity of your decision to pursue a career in medicine. You will have an opportunity to observe trained professionals in action and may get a chance to perform simple tasks yourself. You will find out if you feel comfortable in a hospital and around sick people, as well as how well you manage stress. The person to contact at a hospital is the director of Volunteer Services, who coordinates the efforts of volunteers, arranges their assignments, and conducts their orientation and training. While working in a health care facility is not a stated prerequisite for admission, many medical school admission committees prefer that candidates have this experience. It can show committee members that you have tested your career choice and that your commitment has been reinforced.

Research Experience. In the same way as gaining hospital experience can assist in your career decision, research involvement in a laboratory at your college, a medical school, or a medical research institute can help you decide whether you might be interested in pursuing the Ph.D. degree in addition to the M.D. degree. You might pursue research just because it is interesting and will be a good experience. You might pursue research because medicine is a profession that emphasizes problem-solving. Even if you are not interested in pursuing research as a profession, it is important that you understand such concepts as the scientific method, statistical significance, and the experimental process so that you are capable of critically reviewing research reports in the professional literature and using relevant and valid results in your practice.

The Value of Work. Paying jobs unrelated to medicine may give you experience to help you develop better management and interpersonal skills. Jobs that require considerable contact with the public, for example, can help you develop interaction modes useful in patient care. Jobs that involve management of both work and personnel help develop responsibility and a mature attitude. If you do not have the luxury of volunteering and cannot find a paying job in a hospital, try to use whatever position you find, in a constructive manner, to develop some of these essential "people skills."

Study Abroad. Study Abroad programs can present excellent opportunities for expanded intercultural experiences, both curricular and extracurricular. Medical schools tend to regard Study Abroad participation favorably. However, most schools prefer that the required science coursework, if taken abroad, be strictly comparable to science courses taught in the United States. To avoid the risk of ambiguous interpretation of your academic report, it is a good idea to take all of the required premedical courses in the U.S., either before or after going abroad to study. This can be accomplished by completing all courses necessary for the MCAT and taking the MCAT before going abroad for your junior year, or perhaps going abroad and then applying to medical school after your senior year. There are some other possible variations that can be worked out on an individual basis. If possible, you should begin appropriate planning in your freshman year, in consultation with your prehealth advisor, taking into account all aspects of the medical school application and admission process before making your final decision regarding whether and/or when you will study abroad.

The Application

Your application is your first contact with the medical school admissions office staff and with members of the admission committee. It is therefore a good idea to make a positive first impression by preparing a well-organized application.

1. **When and Where to Apply**
    The medical school application process is a complex one, typically 14 or 15 months in length. The timing of the medical school application is therefore an important consideration. Those who want to begin medical school in the year they graduate from college will apply during the summer between their junior and senior college years. As a general rule, the earlier you apply in the application cycle, the better off you will be. AMCAS (American Medical College Application Service, the central application service for allopathic medical schools) will accept applications beginning on or about June 1, although applicants may begin preparing their online applications on

or about May 1. Consult the MSAR for application dates for those schools that have alternate application processes (e.g., the public medical schools located in Texas).

The majority of medical schools select their students on a "rolling admissions" basis. This means that schools do not wait until all of their application deadlines have passed prior to reviewing and assessing completed applications. Instead they review and accept applicants as their applications and interviews are completed. Thus, if you submit an application later rather than earlier in the application period, fewer seats in the class will be available. The first notification date for regular (non-Early Decision Program) acceptances is October 15; Early Decision Program (EDP) applicants must receive notification of the outcome of their application by October 1. In this scenario, it is possible that some applicants may be accepted before other applicants have even received the results of their August or September MCATs. If you plan to take the MCAT in August or September, it is best to submit all other application materials well before MCAT scores are returned. This approach places you in the best position to have your application reviewed in a timely manner, since your application will be complete at each school once MCAT scores arrive.

You may tend, as many applicants do, to treat medical school application as a one-shot, "do-or-die" situation, based on the assumption that you must be enrolled in medical school immediately after you graduate from college. Medical schools do not care how many years you have spent out of, or away from, school, as long as your academic record, MCAT scores, and other application materials are acceptable to them when you actually apply. There are favorable statistics for those persons who apply after their senior year, as well as for those who apply or reapply to medical school following college graduation. If you took the MCAT only once and did not do as well as you might have hoped, or if your senior year grades would raise your GPA to a more competitive level, you might contemplate waiting to make your first medical school application until after you have completed your college education.

2. **Early Decision Program**
   The Early Decision Program (EDP) is available at many medical schools. This allows an applicant to file an application to a single medical school well before the usual deadline (the deadline for submission of an EDP application is August 1) and to receive a decision from that school promptly (by October 1). If you plan to apply as an EDP candidate, you must take the MCAT no later than the spring of the year in which you apply. If accepted, you agree not to apply to any other schools. If not accepted, you are immediately placed in the regular applicant pool at that school, and you will be able to apply immediately to any other schools of interest. It is quite possible to be denied admission as an EDP candidate and then be accepted during the regular admissions process at the same school. One disadvantage of the EDP is that, if you are not accepted via EDP to the one school to which you applied, your application to other schools will be delayed until that school notifies you of its decision or October 1, at the latest. If accepted, however, you are free to concentrate on your studies during your senior year and/or consider Study Abroad programs or other options.

   You should make an EDP application only to a school that you would be pleased to attend. You should understand that you will probably be competitive for EDP only if your credentials match those of the members of the previous year's entering class at that school. This information for individual medical schools is available in the Medical School Admission Requirements (MSAR) publication.

3. **Deferred Matriculation**
   Many medical schools allow accepted applicants to delay matriculation for one year and will reserve a place for them in the next year's entering class. Each participating school has a policy identifying legitimate reasons for seeking deferred matriculation, and policies vary from school to school. A school's policies on deferred admission are easily determined by consulting the two-page description in MSAR. Depending on individual school policies, you will either be required to attend the school that granted the deferral the following year or you will

be permitted to make application to other schools in the interim. It is therefore extremely important, if you are considering the option of deferred matriculation, that you consult with the individual schools to which you are applying for additional information and that that you not sign any deferred matriculation contract until you are certain about any and all possible conditions.

4. **State Residency Considerations**

When deciding where to apply to medical school, a sensible place to begin is with the latest edition of the MSAR. Included in the descriptions of each medical school are data concerning the number of applicants and matriculants who are state residents and out-of-state candidates. State residency is an important determinant of your chances for medical school acceptance at all public and some private schools. Public medical schools give preferential treatment to residents of their own state; some do not even consider out-of-state residents for admission. If a state has a policy of restricting its class to its own state residents, do not waste your time and money applying there if you are not a resident of that state.

Most private medical schools recruit from the national pool of applicants, rather than primarily from their state pool. At many private schools, however, preferential treatment is also given to in-state residents for a percentage of the class because these schools also receive support from state tax revenues. Some private schools are highly competitive in terms of applicants' GPA and MCAT scores. Other private schools are somewhat less competitive. Check the MSAR for information about selection factors, tuition costs, and the breakdown on state of legal residence. In the MSAR, you will also be able to determine how many resident and non-resident applicants make application to each school, how many are interviewed, and how many actually enter in the first-year class. Ascertain that schools of interest to you do not have special requirements. MSAR also provides information of interest to potential applicants whose states do not have a medical school. In these instances, special arrangements have frequently been made by state governments with medical schools in neighboring states.

Before making final decisions, check with your premedical advisor, who understands the "track record" of your school and the best chances of acceptance for an applicant with your credentials. It is no surprise that once a medical school has admitted some students from a particular institution and has been pleased with their performance, there is a greater likelihood that students from that school will be accepted in the future. If this is the case for your college, you need to be aware of it.

Wherever you apply and to however many schools you apply, include the public schools in your state of legal residence in your application plans. If you are genuinely interested in attending a public school outside your own state, the Early Decision Program may be a good strategy. However, it is good idea to check with individual schools about their EDP policies; some require that EDP candidates be state residents, while a smaller number require EDP candidates to be non-residents.

5. **AMCAS: The Centralized Application Service**

The American Medical College Application Service (AMCAS) is a non-profit, centralized application processing service sponsored by the Association of American Medical Colleges (AAMC). For the 2008 entering class, 124 medical schools and programs will participate in AMCAS, including the M.D./Ph.D. programs at the University of Texas Southwestern Medical School at Dallas, the University of Texas Medical School at Houston, and the University of Texas Medical Branch at Galveston. The M.D. programs at other medical schools (i.e., the public medical schools in Texas, the University of Missouri-Kansas City School of Medicine, and the University of North Dakota School of Medicine and Health Sciences) have alternate application processes. Information about these processes can be found in MSAR. (Note: The public medical schools in Texas use a centralized application of their own, the Texas Medical and Dental School Application Service, www.utsystem.edu/tmdsas) (See Resources).

In applying to AMCAS-participating schools you will submit only one preliminary set of application forms and transcripts, regardless of the number of schools to which you apply; these must be submitted to AMCAS. AMCAS is an entirely Web-based application, accessed at: www.aamc.org/amcas. On this website, you will find links to key steps in initiating an application, an application worksheet that previews the application content, an application timeline, important frequently asked questions (FAQs), and other resources to assist you with the application, including an instruction booklet in PDF format.

You must arrange for a complete set of official transcripts to be forwarded to AMCAS by the registrar of every postsecondary school at which you have ever been registered. Be aware that some institutions take a long time to process transcripts, and you may need to follow up to be certain that all transcripts have actually been sent. In order to fill out the Academic Record portion of the application, you will find it useful to have your own copies of your transcripts, since that is the order in which AMCAS requires the courses be entered.

AMCAS uses your transcripts to verify the courses and grades you have entered on your application; AMCAS also will transmit your MCAT scores to all schools designated by you. Once processing has been completed, the application is sent to all schools designated on your AMCAS form. You receive a notice indicating that this has been done. At this point, AMCAS is finished with your application; from now on, you are in communication with each individual school. No supplemental application materials, such as letters of evaluation or updated information, are sent to AMCAS; they should be sent to the individual medical school. Based on school policies, schools may send you a supplemental application and request an additional application fee, as well as some supporting documents. Once you have received supplemental application materials, the process of applying is similar for both AMCAS and non-AMCAS schools.

A section of the AMCAS application, the Personal Comments section, appears to puzzle many applicants because it is so unstructured. This is a very important component of the application. Applicants should consider carefully how they wish to present themselves in the Personal Comments section. This is your first opportunity to inform an admissions office staff person or admission committee member about yourself: who you are, how you decided upon a medical career, what challenges you have overcome on your path to medical school, your unique characteristics and abilities, and personal experiences that have had a significant impact on your life and career choice. Try to be positive and confident in this section, without appearing arrogant or overconfident. Include concrete examples of your accomplishments, when appropriate, without appearing boastful. It is frequently a good idea to compose your Personal Comments section, then put it aside for a few days before rereading, evaluating, and possibly editing it. The final version should be very carefully checked for spelling, punctuation, grammar, and organization. Keep a hard copy of your Personal Comments section for your own records. It is never appropriate to leave the Personal Comments section blank!

6. **Follow Up**

   To keep your records organized for all schools to which you have applied, set up a separate folder for each medical school, with a checklist for each of the items that you are expected to supply to each school. Medical schools send you complete information regarding the supporting documents they require; these items should be checked off as they are sent. Photocopy documents that are difficult to replace. Most medical schools send to applicants an acknowledgment that the application file has been completed. If you do not receive such notice, you may wish to call the school's admissions office to inquire as to the status of your file.

   It is your responsibility to see that your file is complete at each medical school to which you have applied. While supplementary materials differ for each school, they typically include faculty evaluations (or a composite prehealth committee letter). It is suggested that you supply the number of letters requested and not inundate the admission committee with more than it has requested.

New transcripts of your college coursework should be sent by the registrar's office to those schools at which your application is pending, if the new grades are higher than those on your initial application. Many schools will require grade reports for academic work completed during the application cycle. A personal note along with photocopies of the new grade report will usually suffice. A final official copy of your transcript will be required only after acceptance.

Finally, a number of medical schools require a recent passport size picture as a component of their supplementary application materials. Photos are also needed for MCAT registration. These photographs help to identify you at interviews and will later be used to confirm your identity at the time of matriculation.

Acceptance

1. **What You Can Expect from the Medical Schools**
   AAMC-member medical schools agree to abide by a uniform set of recommendations to govern the process of accepting first-year students. These are sometime referred to as the admission "traffic rules." Accordingly, medical schools agree not to inform candidates of acceptance prior to October 15, except for EDP applicants who will be informed of the outcome of their EDP application by October 1. By March 30, each school is required to have issued a number of acceptances equal to the number of places in the first year class. Prior to May 15, accepted applicants have at least two weeks to respond to an offer of acceptance and can hold acceptance offers from any other schools without penalty. After May 15, medical schools may implement school-specific procedures for accepted applicants who, without adequate explanation, continue to hold one or more places at other schools. These procedures may require applicants to respond to acceptance offers in less than two weeks and/or submit a statement of intent, a deposit, or both. The acceptance deposit should not exceed $100, and it should be refundable until May 15. After June 1, any school that plans to make an acceptance offer to an applicant already known to have been accepted by another school for that entering class should ensure that the other school is advised of this offer at the time that the offer is made. Once accepted applicants have enrolled in medical school or have begun an orientation period immediately prior to enrollment, no additional acceptances may be offered the student by another medical school.

   A complete statement of the "AAMC Recommendations for Medical School Admission Officers" can be found on the AAMC website at: www.aamc.org/students/applying/policies/admissionofficers.htm.

2. **What the Medical Schools Expect from You**
   In a letter of acceptance, medical schools will tell you how much time you have to respond to their offer, as well as any other conditions of acceptance. They expect you to respond to their offer in writing, whether you accept or decline, within the time period they designate.

   Your prompt decision and response to the notification process is important to you and other applicants, as well as to the medical schools where you have been accepted.

   AAMC-member medical schools have also developed a set of admission "traffic rules" for applicants. Applicants are expected to engage in timely communication with schools and to notify schools promptly when there are changes in their contact information. When applicants will be unavailable for an extended period of time, they are expected to identify a responsible party with authority to make decisions on their behalf. Applicants are expected to respond promptly to interview invitations. They are reminded of the importance of getting an early start on their financial aid applications. In addition, after May 15 each year, applicants are only allowed to hold a single acceptance. However, they are permitted to remain on any alternate (waiting) lists that they wish to continue to consider until the time that they matriculate at a medical school or begin the school's orientation immediately prior to matriculation. When an applicant has matriculated at a medical school or has begun an orientation period immediately prior to matriculation, he/she must withdraw any applications from consideration at all other schools at which they remain active until that time.

A complete statement of the "AAMC Recommendations for Medical School Applicants" can be found on the AAMC website at: www.aamc.org/students/applying/policies/applicants.htm.

3. **Multiple Acceptances**

Medical schools expect you to accept the first school that offers you a place. The suggested procedure is as follows: after you receive your first acceptance, rank the schools to which you have applied in order of preference. Send a letter of withdrawal to all schools on your list that are lower than the school to which you have been accepted. As you receive each new acceptance either accept it or reject it, on the basis of how that school compares with the school where you are already holding a seat, and withdraw from any schools that are lower on your list. If you accept the offer, you are still free to accept an offer from a higher priority school if you later receive an offer from that school. When you receive an acceptance from your first-choice school, withdraw from all other schools. In other words, applicants should hold no more than one medical school place at any time, although the medical school at which that place is held may change.

Usually the only legitimate reason to hold two or more acceptances at any one time involves the question of financial aid. If the financial aid package offered will determine where you can attend medical school, you may wait until you receive this information before relinquishing your alternate acceptances. Applicants are expected to have reduced the number of seats they are holding to one school and to withdraw from all other schools from which acceptances have been received immediately after May 15. They may, however, maintain their applications at those higher priority schools from which they have not received a decision (i.e., remain on the alternate list) after May 15.

4. **The Alternate List**

Each year, medical schools "lose" some of those applicants to whom they have offered seats as those applicants choose to attend other medical schools. To cope with this eventuality, schools keep lists of candidates who would be acceptable to them if they had an available place. This list is usually referred to as the "alternate list" or "waiting list." After all initial acceptances have been sent out, applicants are informed if they are on the alternate list. Unfortunately, there is no uniformity concerning wait-listing; every school appears to have its own preferred method. Nevertheless, there are several broad categories into which procedures fall.

At some schools, the alternate list appears to be "written in stone." The list is ranked by admission committee members, and alternates are accepted from the list in strict numerical order. There is generally nothing an applicant can do to enhance his or her position on the list. At schools where alternate lists are not ranked, the lists are reviewed periodically and some movement may be possible.

Those schools that divide their waiting lists into sections (for example, "upper," "middle," or "lower third") usually inform applicants where they are on the list and give them guidelines as to their chance of acceptance from the list based on prior years' experience.

5. **School Procedures**

All schools inform candidates when they have been placed on their alternate list. The letter may or may not contain further elaboration of the school's policy. The answers to such questions as how long the list is, where you stand on the list, and how many applicants have been accepted from the alternate list in the past depends on each school. The best way to have questions answered is to speak to a staff member in the school's admissions office and/or to your prehealth advisor.

Acceptance from the alternate list will come in a letter or perhaps in a phone call from the admissions office, sometimes as late as immediately before the academic year begins. It is wise for applicants to notify the admissions office of the address, telephone number, and email address at which they can be reached during the summer months. If students plan to travel during the summer, they should have a back-up number available where messages can be left.

6. **Candidates' Responses**

When you learn that you have been placed on an alternate list and you are interested in attending that school, the first thing to do is respond to the school in writing. Let the school know that you want to keep your place on the alternate list and that you are interested in the school. Next, find out as much as possible about your status by calling the medical school admissions office (without being a pest) and by speaking with your prehealth advisor. Medical schools do not mind your contacting them when you have been named an alternate; if anything, it is considered a sign of your continuing interest in the school. More importantly, you should ascertain whether or not there is anything you can do that will influence your chances of acceptance. Items meaningful at some schools are your grade report from the past semester or summer session, any honors you received after your application was submitted, publications, or new experiences that might be relevant to your application.

If you are on several medical schools' alternate lists, your chances of being accepted by one of the schools increases. If you have not received an acceptance, but have been placed on an alternate list, it is a good idea to make tentative plans for the following year, should you not ultimately receive an acceptance. Psychologically, it is better to be involved in some positive action rather than merely fantasizing about receiving an acceptance letter each day the mail is delivered. Should you actually receive that letter, you will probably have very little difficulty in adjusting. If you should not, then you have alternative plans already in place. Remember, you were very close to being accepted, and the probability for success on a reapplication is usually good, especially if you strengthen your application in some significant way during the intervening year.

Special Programs

1. **Joint Degree Programs**

   A. **M.D./Ph.D. Degree Programs**

   A complete listing of joint and combined degree programs at medical schools is available on the AAMC website at: services.aamc.org/currdir/start.cfm. These programs are sometimes administered collaboratively by the medical school and the graduate school at an institution. They provide students with the opportunity to pursue both the M.D. and Ph.D. degrees in an integrated program. At present, such programs have been identified at the majority of medical schools in the United States. Depending on the program, enrollment can vary from two or three to over one hundred students. The size of the program relative to the overall enrollment in the school is another way in which programs differ. In some schools, the proportion of students pursuing combined degree programs is large, while at other schools it is very small.

   Several programs have been in operation for decades, when the National Institutes of Health established the Medical Scientist Training Program (MSTP) to encourage M.D./Ph.D. education by providing funds to medical schools to support students enrolled in M.D./Ph.D. programs, while others have been more recently established. The National Institute of General Medical Sciences maintains websites that contain general information about the Medical Scientist Training Program (www.nigms.nih.gov/training/mstp.html) and about institutions that have received MSTP funding (www.nigms.nih.gov/Training/Mechanisms/NRSA/InstPredoc/PredocInst-MSTP.htm).

Students in M.D./Ph.D. programs are frequently, although not always, provided with financial support, a practical necessity in light of the six to eight years of enrollment required. In addition to federal funding available for student support, funding often occurs via the medical school and/or graduate department. Several programs have received significant endowments from outside private sources.

M.D./Ph.D. programs vary with respect to the fields in which Ph.D.s are offered and the number of different Ph.D. programs available. Typically, the Ph.D. can be pursued in a variety of the basic sciences, including, but not limited to, anatomy, biochemistry, cell biology, developmental biology, genetics, immunology, microbiology, molecular biology, neurosciences, pathology, and pharmacology. Medical schools that are a component of research universities are likely to enable students to pursue the Ph.D. in graduate departments of the university and are, therefore, also likely to be able to offer more diverse areas of doctoral specialization. Reflecting the "high-tech" nature of modern medicine, several schools offer combined degree programs in medicine and the engineering sciences, physics, or computer science. In responding to the need to educate physicians to deal with the social and economic forces affecting medicine, some M.D./Ph.D. programs enable students to pursue their doctoral education in the social and behavioral sciences and the humanities, in disciplines such as anthropology, economics, philosophy, and psychology.

Students typically apply to joint degree programs at the same time they apply to the medical school, and most programs have a separate admission process in which admission to the medical school and admission to the graduate program are independent decisions. Some programs also accept applications from first- and second-year medical students at their school. The sequence of study generally begins with the medical curriculum, but there is variation and general agreement among programs that flexibility in scheduling is desirable.

Selection criteria for M.D./Ph.D. programs are generally identical to those for medical school, although higher standards may be applied to grades and test scores because of the demanding nature of combined degree education. An important additional criterion is research ability, usually evaluated on the basis of an applicant's previous experience, letters of recommendation, and discussion in interviews. If you are seeking information about M.D./Ph.D. programs, you should consider importance of research to your overall professional goals. If your primary interest is in clinical medicine, and you are considering combined degree programs because you are interested in a second field or because it might be a good "backup," the investment of an additional four years of education is probably not wise. The commitment to research must be very strong to provide a rationale and motivation to pursue both the M.D. and Ph.D. degrees. There are, of course, excellent opportunities for carrying out high-level research in clinical settings.

Alumni of M.D./Ph.D. programs have joined the leadership ranks in academic medicine, in government and independent research laboratories, in the corporate sector, and in public and private voluntary organizations. Many are already active in determining public policy, and it can be anticipated that those with scholarly training in the social sciences and humanities will be nationally prominent in this sphere. It is expected that there will be a ongoing need for physicians with advanced research skills and for those with the sophisticated understanding of the socio-economic forces impinging upon health care that graduate training provides.

B. **Other Joint Degree Programs**

It also is possible to pursue a medical degree in conjunction with another graduate or professional degree: M.P.H., M.B.A., J.D., or other Master's degree (e.g., in Education). In 2007, 21 schools were identified that offered M.D./J.D. programs. An additional 49 schools sponsored M.D./M.B.A. degree programs. Seventy-one schools report the availability of M.D./M.P.H. programs. A listing of all available M.D./graduate programs can be found on the AAMC website at: services.aamc.org/currdir/start.cfm.

2. **Baccalaureate-M.D. Programs**

Approximately one-quarter of medical schools sponsor joint baccalaureate/M.D. programs with either their own undergraduate institutions or other schools in their geographic region. The nature of these programs varies greatly, with a small number providing accelerated programs leading to both degrees in a six to seven-year time period and one program providing intensive study in medicine and engineering in nine years. Most programs provide students with the opportunity to complete their undergraduate and medical studies in seven or eight years. Typically, such programs offer the baccalaureate degree after completion of the first year of medical school. A complete listing of such programs can be found in MSAR. If you are interested in pursuing such a program, consult with your health professions advisor. Be aware, however, that many of these medical school programs are, in fact, restricted to students from their own undergraduate schools or others with which they have joint programs.

Schools and Colleges of Medicine

A comprehensive listing of all allopathic medical schools in the United States and Canada, as well as information about various criteria used to compare medical schools (e.g., amount of research funding from the National Institutes of Health, tuition and fees) can be found on the AAMC website at: www.aamc.org/medicalschools.htm.

Resources

1. *Medical School Admission Requirements* (MSAR). Published annually (in late spring) by AAMC. This book contains the latest available information on selection factors and the credentials of accepted applicants for each medical school in the U.S. and Canada. The latest edition should be consulted by every student during the time the decision is being made as to where to apply. It may be available for purchase at your university bookstore, commercial bookstore, and online, or it may be ordered from the AAMC (www.aamc.org/msar). It may also be available for in-office use at your school's Health Professions Advising Office.

2. *MCAT Essentials.* Available as a PDF document from the AAMC website at: www.aamc.org/mcat.

3. Various AAMC print and electronic publications of interest to applicants. Available on the AAMC website at: www.aamc.org/publications; click on "Applicants."

4. AAMC Careers in Medicine Program online career planning program. Available on the AAMC website at: www.aamc.org/careersinmedicine.

5. FIRST. The AAMC has recently instituted a comprehensive program on pre-medical, medical, and post-graduate physician indebtedness entitled FIRST (Financial Instruments, Resources, Services, and Tools) which provides useful information and economic calculators for all levels of physicians in their careers. The website is at www.aamc.org/programs/first.

6. *AAMC Curriculum Directory.* A comprehensive website containing various searchable databases of information about medical school curricula, institutional characteristics, and combined degree programs. Available on the AAMC website at: services.aamc.org/currdir/start.cfm.

7. The AAMC TomorrowsDoctors website: www.tomorrowsdoctors.org. A comprehensive website for those considering a career in medicine, those applying to medical school, medical students, and residents.

8. The website of the AspiringDocs.org program: www.aspiringdocs.org. Information for persons from groups underrepresented in medicine who are considering a career in the medical profession.

9. *The New Physician.* A monthly magazine published by the American Medical Student Association, 1910 Association Drive, Reston, VA 22091 (www.amsa.org).

    Membership in AMSA for premedical students is available for a fee which includes a subscription to The New Physician, a good source of information about trends in medical education, financial aid, and other timely topics.

10. *Write for Success: Preparing a Professional School Application.* A booklet by Evelyn Jackson and Harold Bardo, both at the School of Medicine, Southern Illinois University, written specifically to help applicants to medical school present themselves in the best possible light. Published by NAAHP, Inc., P.O. Box 1518, Champaign IL 61824-1518; 217/355-0063; fax: 217/355-1287; www.naahp.org.

11. *Interviewing for Health Professions Schools.* A booklet offering concise, comprehensive information that helps students prepare for the interview. Published by NAAHP, Inc. (See address above.)

12. The website of the Bureau of Health Professions, Health Resources Services Administration: www.bhpr.hrsa.gov.

13. The website of the American Medical College Application Service (AMCAS): www.aamc.org/amcas. Information about making application to AMCAS-participating schools and programs.

14. The website of the American Medical Association: www.ama-assn.org. Information about becoming a physician; preparing for, applying to, and paying for medical school; and choosing a specialty.

15. The website of the Texas Medical and Dental Schools Application Service: www.utsystem.edu/tmdsas. Information about making application to the public medical schools in the state of Texas.

DENTISTRY (D.M.D., D.D.S.)

General Description of the Profession

Dentistry is a profession that combines science and technology with helping people to enhance and maintain their oral health. As health care practitioners, dentists diagnose, treat, and help prevent diseases, injuries and malformations of the teeth and mouth. They improve a patient's appearance by using a variety of cosmetic dental procedures; perform surgical procedures such as implants, tissue grants and extractions; educate patients on how to better care of their teeth and prevent oral disease; teach future dentists and dental hygienists; and perform research directed to developing new treatment methods and improving oral health.

The majority of the more than 175,000 professionally active dentists are private practitioners. Most dentists practice in an office setting, typically in a solo practice with an average of five employees. The majority enter a practice immediately after receiving a doctoral degree in dentistry, either a Doctor of Dental Surgery (D.D.S) or a Doctor of Dental Medicine (D.M.D) (there is no difference between the two degrees).

About 82% of dentists in the U.S. are general practitioners. The remaining 18% of dentists are involved in one of the nine dental specialties recognized by the American Dental Association, which require additional education after the D.M.D. or D.D.S. The nine specialties are: (1) orthodontics and dentofacial orthopedics — the treatment of problems relating to dental development, missing teeth, and other abnormalities affecting both normal function and appearance; (2) oral and maxillofacial surgery — the diagnostic and operative services dealing with disease, injuries, and defects in the jaw and related structures; (3) endodontics — the diagnosis, prevention and treatment of diseases of the pulp and other dental tissues that affect the vitality of the teeth; (4) periodontics — the diagnosis and treatment of diseases that affect the oral mucous membranes and other soft tissues that surround and support the teeth; (5) pediatric dentistry — the treatment of children and adolescents; (6) prosthodontics — the replacement of missing natural teeth with fixed or removable substitutes; (7) oral and maxillofacial pathology — the provision of diagnostic and consultative biopsy services to dentists and physicians; (8) dental public health — the control and prevention of dental disease through organized community efforts, and (9) oral and maxillofacial radiology, a specialty area using the images and data produced by all modalities of radiant energy to diagnose and manage diseases, disorders and conditions of the oral and maxillofacial regions.

The career outlook for new dental practitioners is good. New dentists are needed in private practice, as teachers and researchers and in public health, because large numbers of dentists are projected to retire in the next 20 years. Increasing numbers of older adults are keeping their teeth longer; there is a greater awareness of oral health care, including links between oral and overall heath, and there is a greatly increased demand for cosmetic services such as bonding and veneers. Technological advances such as digital radiology, laser systems, computer designed restorations and informatics allow dentists to provide treatment more effectively.

The Decision to Pursue Dentistry as a Career

Most students (70%) make the decision to attend dental school either during or after college, thus making it imperative that health professions advisors be cognizant of the profession and admission procedures. Surveys of graduating dental students indicate that the about 30% entered college with the intention of attending dental school. Factors influencing decisions to pursue a career in dentistry include the ability to deliver healthcare, awareness of emerging research about connections between oral health and overall health, and lifestyle considerations such as the flexibility to balance a professional and a personal life.

Dentistry provides an opportunity for an excellent income (in the top 5% among U.S. citizens), a satisfying professional career, and time for a personal life. Recent surveys indicate that the mean annual net income of general dentists in private practice is nearly $200,000 and over $300,000 for specialists. Many dentists enjoy the independence and autonomy of owning their own practices, including the flexibility of determining their practice hours. Dentists in private practice benefit from opportunities to establish one-on-one relationships with patients over time. Dentistry is viewed by the public as one of the most trusted and ethical professions in the U.S.

Aptitude for the sciences, the ability to visually perceive depth, color and shape, and possession of manual dexterity are essential to practice dentistry. Because most dentists provide care in private practice settings, knowledge of business and personal finance is also helpful.

While only 16% of all professionally active U.S. dentists are female, more women are entering dental school than ever before. In 2007, women comprised 45% of students enrolled in US dental schools. It is anticipated that by 2020, approximately 30% of all professionally active dentists will be women.

Approximately 7% of all professionally active U.S. dentists are underrepresented minorities (3.5% African American, 3.5% Hispanic/Latino, <.01% Native American/American Indian). Dental education is challenged to build a dental workforce that reflects the nation's diversity. To achieve a more balanced workforce to adequately serve the public, the dental profession seeks to increase the number of underrepresented minorities, individuals from disadvantaged backgrounds and individuals from underserved areas.

Planning a Program of Study

General Information

As of December 2008, there are 57 dental schools in the U.S that are fully accredited by the Commission on Dental Accreditation of the American Dental Association. Plans are underway for several new dental schools to begin accepting students within the next few years.

The best references about dental school programs of study are the ADEA *Official Guide to Dental Schools* and ADEA's *Opportunities for Minority Students in U.S. Dental Schools*. Updated annually, the *Official Guide* provides descriptive information and statistics from each of the U.S. and Canadian dental schools. *Opportunities for Minority Students in U.S. Dental Schools* features profiles of minority dentists and includes additional information about summer enrichment programs, postbaccalaureate programs and other opportunities. Both publications are provided free of charge to NAAHP members; additional copies may be ordered through the American Dental Education Association (ADEA) at www.adea.org.

Admission requirements to the dental schools vary by school. It is important for pre-dental students to be aware of the specific requirements of the schools to which they may apply. The majority require a minimum of 8 semester hours (or 12 quarter hours) each of biology, general chemistry, organic chemistry and physics. Increasingly, some dental schools seek applicants who have completed additional upper-level courses such as biochemistry, microbiology and genetics. Many also require courses in English, mathematics and social sciences.

Most dental schools give preference to candidates who will have earned a baccalaureate degree prior to matriculation in dental school. Although a minimum of two years of preprofessional study is required by most dental schools prior to admission, typically less than 1% of the class matriculating has such minimum preparation.

Choice of Undergraduate Major

The majority of dental students majored in the biological and natural sciences. However, it is not necessary to major in a science. Dental admission committees do not look for a particular undergraduate major as long as applicants have completed course requirements and demonstrate sufficient academic preparation. Other academic majors of pre-dental students include business, social sciences, engineering, architecture and the humanities.

The Admissions Process

Factors Evaluated by Admission Committees

Dental schools use admission committees for selection of entering classes. The size and composition of committees vary from school to school, but they are typically composed of clinical and basic science faculty, and in many schools, dental students, alumni and practicing dentists. Schools seek to select applicants exhibiting evidence of high intellectual competence, demonstrated knowledge and interest in the profession, cultural sensitivity, and personal traits to relate compassionately to patients. Communication skills, leadership ability, good character, motivation and knowledge of the field of dentistry are all evaluated by admissions committees.

The strength of academic preparation, as demonstrated by courses completed, grades earned, and DAT scores very are important factors in admissions decisions. However, other factors can influence admissions decisions. Many admissions committees encourage the "whole file" review of applicants, considering factors such as challenges faced in pursuing a college education, improving performance, and successfully balancing academics, work and extracurricular activities.

1. **Academic Record**

The undergraduate record is usually considered the single most important factor in admissions decisions. The academic record includes the cumulative grade point averages, courses completed, academic rigor, and trends in performance (i.e., improving grades during the undergraduate program). A strong undergraduate academic record is considered evidence of both ability and academic preparedness. Grades are not evaluated alone, but in the context of the total academic program, along with such factors as employment, participation in extracurricular activities and other demands on study time. Applicants with special interests, i.e., research, teaching, commitment to serving underserved or disadvantaged populations, etc. are often favorably considered.

2. **The Standardized Test (DAT)**

The Dental Admission Test (DAT) is required by all U.S. dental schools. This test measures general academic ability, comprehension of scientific information, and perceptual ability.

Predental students are strongly encouraged to prepare for the DAT. Good DAT scores can significantly enhance an applicant's chances of being seriously considered for admission.

The DAT is administered by the American Dental Association as a computerized test at Prometric Test Centers and can be taken at the time of the applicant's choosing. Candidates applying for the DAT must submit an application and fee payment to the Dental Admission Testing Program (see Resources). Candidates receive instruction for making test arrangements following the processing of their materials. The DAT fee covers the cost of forwarding score transcripts to five dental schools, a copy to the applicant, and a copy to the health professions advisor.

Candidates are required to submit a new application and fee for each re-examination and must wait at least *90 days* before retaking the DAT. The results of the four most recent DAT's are released on the official report of scores and forwarded to dental schools. Effective in 2007, candidates may take the DAT no more than three times; exceptions can be granted in unusual situations. Refer to the DAT website for more information.

The candidate receives unofficial DAT scores immediately after completing the four tests in the DAT battery. Dental Schools (selected on the candidate's application to receive DAT scores) will receive them approximately three weeks after the testing date. Predental advisors receive Reports of DAT performance quarterly.

The multiple choice examination takes just over a half day to complete and consists of four examinations: *survey of natural sciences, perceptual ability, reading comprehension, and quantitative reasoning.*

The material tested in the sciences is at the introductory level, i.e., topics that would normally be covered in a rigorous one-year introductory sequence in general chemistry, organic chemistry and biology. It is not necessary, or typically beneficial, to study from advanced textbooks in a subject. Test questions are often posed so that the application of general principles is stressed more than regurgitation of facts. The facts must be known, but the candidate must also be able to apply these facts to solve problems.

The *DAT Program Guide,* located on the ADA's website, contains an outline of the topics to be tested. A careful review of these areas is recommended. The four areas are:
- *Survey of Natural Sciences* (longest test) includes biology, general chemistry and organic chemistry
- *Reading Comprehension* (taken from basic science subjects usually with a dental emphasis)
- *Quantitative Ability* (math problems that test mathematical reasoning — does not require calculus or trigonometry)
- *Perceptual Ability* (two- and three-dimensional spatial problem solving)

It should be emphasized that there are no "tricks" or "strategies" that can substitute for knowledge of the subject, particularly in the science sections.

The Examinee Guide, sample DAT and registration materials are available at www.ada.org. Candidates may register for the test online. A tutorial is also available that familiarizes the candidate with the process of taking the computerized DAT, as well as a sample DAT test. Beginning in 2007, in the event an examinee has a dispute with the testing program, the candidate agrees to submit the dispute to arbitration if dissatisfied with the outcome of the program's standard appeal process.

Typical questions and answers regarding the DAT:

What is an acceptable DAT score?
This varies with the dental schools. The latest edition of the ADEA *Official Guide to Dental Schools* should be reviewed to determine DAT scores and GPAs that are competitive at a particular school. Applicants with lower GPA's who score well on the DAT can significantly enhance their competitiveness for admission to dental school.

What can be done to assure acceptable scores on the DAT?
Experience has shown that an organized and systematic review of the topics tested on the DAT can result in a considerable, sometimes dramatic, improvement in DAT scores. Applicants are strongly encouraged to be familiar with both the format and the subject content of the test before sitting for the test.

Are sample tests available?
A sample test is available at the ADA website, www.ada.org.

There are a number of companies that offer review courses for the DAT. The NAAHP does not endorse any of these commercial enterprises, but the pros and cons of enrolling in such courses are discussed elsewhere in this book. It is not necessary to take a commercial review course in order to score well on the DAT. Many disciplined students review the DAT sample test materials and prepare by reviewing their personal notes and textbooks.

No matter what method is chosen to review the material for the DAT, the candidate should begin several weeks before the test date with a specific block of time set aside to study, preferably daily. It is much better to study on a daily basis rather than attempt to review huge blocks of material at a time. Old notes and textbooks are particularly valuable resources since the emphasis should be on reviewing familiar concepts rather than learning new material.

Applicants are encouraged to check the registration form that will allow distribution of test scores to their health professions advisors. To maintain a strong advising program, these scores must be available to the advisor, both for use in advising individual students and for the preparation of summary reports. Individual scores are protected by federal legislation (The Family Educational Rights and Privacy Act) and are never released without written authorization by the student concerned.

3. **Letters of Evaluation**

Most dental schools require three or four letters of evaluation (or recommendation) to consider an application complete. There are three general methods used to compile and submit letters of evaluation: 1) a predental committee report/letter, 2) a composite letter submitted by a health profession advising office, and 3) individual letters of evaluation sent to the application service (or directly to the dental school). A pre-dental committee report generally consists of an evaluation of the applicant that is a composite of opinions of the members of the committee; it is sometimes composed after an in-depth interview with the applicant; supporting letters of evaluation from other faculty are frequently appended. A composite letter consists of a collection of individual letters of evaluation that are collected by a health professions advisor or advising office and supplied to the application service under a cover letter from the advising office. If these services are not available, applicants may opt to have letters of evaluation submitted directly to the application service.

Most dental schools prefer at least three faculty evaluation letters, with two from science faculty. A letter of support from a dentist with whom the applicant has shadowed and/or discussed the profession is strongly encouraged. Admissions committees seek insight into an applicant's ability and motivation to pursue advanced education, special experiences or qualities, special challenges the applicant may have overcome, awareness of issues in the profession, and the potential to adhere to a strong code of professional conduct.

4. **The Interview**

Most dental schools require the individuals they are seriously considering for admission to participate in a personal interview. Interview formats vary by dental school, from traditional one-on-one interviews with members of the Admissions Committees to small group interviews where groups of applicants discuss a particular ethical dilemma or related issue. Applicants invited for interview are usually provided information about the type of interview in which they will be expected to participate, either through their invitation notification, or by being directed to special websites.

Applicants should be prepared to discuss their motivation for a career in dentistry as well as their personal and professional goals, and possess awareness of oral health issues. Participating in mock interviews is strongly encouraged.

At many dental schools, the interview process includes opportunities for applicants to tour the school, meet with current students, and learn about special aspects of the program, including financial aid. The interview visit is an opportunity both for the applicant to develop a sense of "fit" with the school and for the Admissions Committee to assess the potential for the applicant to be successful if admitted.

Applicants should anticipate the cost of participating interviews, including travel, hotel stays and a suit or other professional clothing.

5. **Extracurricular Activities and Work Experience**

Extracurricular activities and work experience can enhance an application in many ways: demonstrating commitment to helping others, heightening awareness of oral health issues, serving in leadership positions, and the demonstrating the ability to manage multiple priorities along with academics. Admission committees are much more interested in the demonstration of leadership and genuine commitment over time than they are to an exhaustive list of activities that require one-time or occasional participation. The extent of participation in extracurricular activities will vary by applicant, depending on work and other personal demands.

It is not necessary for extracurricular activities or work experience to occur in a dental setting, although such experiences can be quite valuable. Many dental schools require specified shadowing hours to be documented as a part of the application. Applicants should be encouraged to shadow *general dentists*, taking the time to discuss those qualities they find both most rewarding and least satisfying. Admissions committees seek assurance that the applicant understands the profession.

The Application

1. When and Where to Apply

AADSAS (the Associated American Dental Schools Application Service, www.adea.org, is a centralized application service of the American Dental Education Association (ADEA). As of the 2009 application cycle, 55 dental schools participate in AADSAS, (54 U.S. schools and one Canadian school). Applicants submit a single application to AADSAS; transcripts are verified, grade point averages are calculated, and AADSAS sends a standard applicant packet to each of the dental schools the applicant designates. AADSAS also collects and disseminates letters of evaluation that are submitted on behalf of applicants. As of December 2008, four U.S. dental schools do not participate in AADSAS and candidates must apply to them directly. Texas residents applying to Texas dental schools must utilize the Texas Application Service (www.utsystem.edu/tmdsas).

The online AADSAS application becomes available June 1 for the next entering class. For example, the AADSAS 2010 application cycle begins on June 1, 2009. Each dental school has its own AADSAS application deadlines, which range from September 1 to February 1. Consult the AADSAS application and individual dental school websites for current deadlines.

Applicants are *strongly encouraged to apply early*. Depending on application volume, AADSAS processing takes four to six weeks. Dental schools begin receiving applications in June, and generally begin interviews in August and September. Many — but not all — dental schools have supplemental applications and fees that must be submitted to consider the application complete.

Factors such as residency, mission and location of the dental school can be important factors in the section of dental schools. Applicants are encouraged to become acquainted with the dental schools by reviewing the ADEA *Official Guide to Dental Schools* and dental school websites. Because admission to dental school is competitive, applicants are encouraged to apply to more than one school.

AADSAS applicants can track the status of their applications by monitoring their online AADSAS application. Applicant data is sent to the dental schools electronically and in print format. Refer to the AADSAS website (www.adea.org) for more complete information about application processing.

Acceptance

Dental schools begin sending offers of acceptance, starting December 1. Individuals accepted in December have 45 days to accept their offers of admission; those accepted in January have 30 days to accept offers; those accepted in February 1 or later have 15 days; those accepted after July 15 or two weeks before the start of dental school classes (whichever is sooner) may be asked for an immediate response. Most dental schools require a tuition deposit (often non-refundable) to hold a position in a class. Deposits can vary by school, ranging from $100 to more than $2,000.

Most dental schools develop a wait list or alternate list of candidates who will be considered for admission if a previously confirmed applicant withdraws. The size each school's wait list varies, as does each school's policy of selecting candidates from the wait list. On May 1, dental schools report to AADSAS the names of their confirmed acceptances and AADSAS provides each school with the names of those applicants who hold positions at more than one school. Dental schools may contact such individuals and may rescind an offer of admission if there is no resolution after 15 days.

Special Programs

Many dental schools offer summer enrichment and other programs for pre-dental students from disadvantaged backgrounds and underserved areas. Frequently, these programs are co-sponsored with other health professions or the main university. A listing of programs can be found ADEA *Opportunities for Minority Students in U.S. Dental Schools* (published biennially). For the most up-to-date list of such programs, consult explorehealthcareers.org.

Joint Degree Programs

Joint degree programs provide applicants the opportunity to earn a Master's or Ph.D. degree in combination with their DDS or DMD. These degree programs are particularly appealing to individuals considering a career in academic dentistry, or those who are considering specialty training. Joint degree programs can include Master's and Ph.D. degrees in oral biology and the basic sciences, as well as Master's in Public Health and Master's in Business Administration degrees. Check the ADEA *Official Guide to Dental Schools* for a current listing of schools that offer joint degree programs.

Financing a Dental Education

The best single reference for financial aid for dental students is Chapter 4 of the ADEA *Official Guide to Dental Schools*, Financing Your Dental Education. This chapter includes information about how to apply for financial aid, how financial aid is awarded, and details the various types of financial aid awarded to dental students. Because more than 90% of dental student receive financial aid and because the majority of financial aid to dental students is in the form of student loans, most colleges and universities have financial aid officers — either in the dental school or on the health sciences campus — who work specifically with dental students.

Most dental school websites offer detailed information about costs and financial aid resources at their dental schools. Applicants should initiate contact with the financial aid office early, because types, terms and deadlines for dental student financial aid programs vary.

Schools and Colleges of Dentistry

As of December 2008, there are 57 accredited U.S. dental schools. Several additional dental schools are currently in development and anticipate accepting entering classes in upcoming years. Consult the ADEA website (www.adea.org) for a current list of dental schools and links to their websites.

Resources

1. *ADEA Official Guide to Dental Schools* is published annually (in January-February) by the American Dental Education Association and contains the latest available program descriptions, selection criteria and the credentials of admitted students for each dental school in the U.S. and Canada. The *ADEA Official Guide to Dental Schools* may be purchased online at the ADEA website (www.adea.org) and can also be found in many libraries and health professions advising offices.

2. *Opportunities for Minority Students in U.S. Dental Schools* is available online the American Dental Education Association (www.adea.org) and provides useful information about applying to dental schools, including summer enrichment and post-baccalaureate programs, profiles of minority dental students and dentists, and financial aid information and profiles of each dental school. This publication is widely distributed to college libraries and health professions offices.

3. www.ExploreHealthCareers.org (sponsored by the American Dental Education Association) provides up-to-date information about all health-related occupations including information about summer enrichment programs, special opportunities and post-baccalaureate programs.

4. Dental Admission Test (www.ada.org/prof/ed/testing/dat). Students must register online for the DAT. This site includes a practice test and complete information about registering for and taking the test.

5. Dentistry career information (www.ada.org/goto/careers). Targeted career information for predental students and health advisors on job shadowing, career exploring programs and additional resources.

6. American Student Dental Association (www.asdanet.org): The American Student Dental Association (ASDA) is the largest national student-run organization which protects and advances the rights, interests, and welfare of students pursuing careers in dentistry. It introduces students to lifelong involvement in organized dentistry and provides services, information, education, representation and advocacy.

ASDA's membership includes predental, predoctoral, and international students, as well as associate members who are interested in the field of dentistry. ASDA offers the following publications to keep members informed on the current issues and concerns of dental students:

- *ASDA News*, a monthly newspaper that serves as a platform for dental, association and student news. The newspaper includes association and industry news, chapter events, student columns and advice on clinical board exams, practice management and making the transition from dental school to dental practice.
- *Mouth*, a quarterly journal dedicated to keeping dental students informed of current trends by bringing scientific- and issue-oriented subjects of interest to its readers. The journal's departments include case reports, book reviews, new product announcements, technical quizzes, news briefs, student perspectives and a historical look at dentistry.
- *Getting into Dental School: ASDA's Guide for Predental Students*, a resource guide specifically targeting the needs of predental students and those considering careers in dentistry.
- *Getting Through Dental School: ASDA's Guide for Dental Students*, a resource guide provided to all predoctoral members providing information on scholarships and loans, career paths, board preparation and licensure
- *Guide to Postdoctoral Programs Vol. 1-3*, designed to make the process of comparing graduate programs more efficient and convenient for applicants, the three-volume set contains up-to-date comparative information about advanced education in general dentistry, dental public health, endodontics, general practice residencies, oral and maxillofacial pathology, orthodontics, pediatric dentistry, periodontics and prosthodontics programs.

For further information, contact the American Student Dental Association, 211 East Chicago Avenue, Suite 700, Chicago, Illinois 60611; Phone 312-440-2795; membership@ASDAnet.org; www.asdanet.org.

HEALTH ADMINISTRATION (B.S., M.S., Ph.D.)

General Description of the Profession

Healthcare is a business and, like every other business, it needs good management to keep it running smoothly. The term "healthcare administrator/healthcare manager" applies to those professionals who plan, direct, coordinate, and supervise the delivery of healthcare.

Today, an estimated 100,000 people serve in healthcare management from middle management to CEO positions at organizations that range in size from 1-2 staff members to major international companies employing hundreds of thousands of employees.

The Decision to Pursue a Career in Healthcare Management

You are a caring and compassionate person. You want to make a real difference in the lives of others, and you want to make the world a better place. You are also adaptable and able to think clearly and strategically on complex problems. Most of all, you are drawn to the professionalism, to the application of leadership skills in organizations which can clearly improve the lives of others, and to the challenging mission of healthcare management.

Once you have made the decision to pursue a career in this profession, you need to determine what degree will best prepare you to begin your career and enhance your opportunities in the future. The answer should be a degree from an accredited graduate healthcare management program or a certified undergraduate healthcare management program.*

An accredited or certified healthcare management degree can provide you with both an in depth understanding of the health sector and the essential competencies needed for the practice. When you graduate from a healthcare management program, you are uniquely prepared to manage a broad spectrum of healthcare organizations. At the same time, a healthcare management degree program offers mentoring and field experiences with senior healthcare executives that are rarely duplicated in other degree programs. You gain a competitive advantage both in launching your career and in learning applied competencies that are essential for your success.

Moreover, your accredited or certified degree has earned the highest respect among most healthcare organizations as they recruit for new management talent. You have the advantage of understanding the specialized language, financing, and politics of the healthcare system. Your critical thinking skills in healthcare management and your knowledge of this dynamic and complex sector will provide a significant advantage in your professional preparation.

The career opportunities with a healthcare management degree are expansive and invigorating — including hospital and health systems management, medical groups, pharmaceutical and biotechnology companies, care management organizations, health information technology firms, supply chain companies, government/policy organizations, health insurers, banks, and healthcare management consulting firms. The healthcare management community and program alumni provide you with advancement opportunities and a network of contacts that is invaluable as you progress throughout your career.

Prepare to launch your career in healthcare management by selecting the approach that provides specialized skills and knowledge essential to managing health related organizations — something not available in traditional management programs.

Reasons to Pursue a Career in Healthcare Management

Making a Difference/Social Mission — Decisions made by healthcare executives can help improve life for hundreds, even thousands of people every day. Healthcare executives have a sense of social mission — they deeply care about the people they work with and serve. Further, our hospitals and healthcare organizations provide opportunities for those who want to "do well by doing good."

Career Opportunities — Healthcare is the largest industry in the U.S., and the second largest employer, with more than 11 million jobs. Virtually all new private sector jobs over the past 5 years came from healthcare; and the sector continues to grow faster than most other segments[1]

Furthermore, unlike many traditional management programs, graduates of healthcare management programs can find significant opportunities in areas ranging from small rural communities to large metropolitan areas and throughout the world.

Excellent Earning Potential — Students pursuing healthcare management careers have excellent earning potential. For the most recent figures and information, see the U.S. Bureau of Labor Statistics website at www.bls.gov/oco/ocos014.htm. Senior healthcare executives with more experience and achievements can earn $200,000 or significantly more.

Career Flexibility — An education in healthcare management can take you in many different and exciting directions. In addition to more traditional careers in healthcare management, graduates work in many other areas including: pharmaceutical companies, health insurance companies, management consulting, banks and other financial institutions, long-term care facilities, professional societies and state and Federal agencies.

The core skill set you develop in a healthcare management program provides a competitive advantage within the healthcare sector. In addition, these skills transfer readily across a variety of industries, providing flexibility for non-health sector positions as well.

Management and Advancement Potential — There is an excellent career ladder — and many people also take on roles in different sectors of the field over the course of their careers.

Visible and Valued Role in the Community — Healthcare executives typically are highly respected members of their communities. Hospitals and other healthcare organizations are among the largest employers in many communities and their organizations positively impact the health of the populations they serve and the well-being of their community.

Continual Self Improvement — Healthcare management is a career that values continual self improvement and education, and most employers encourage continued professional development. Many organizations often support tuition remission or in-service training for new skills. Innovation and continuous learning will be a part of the job from the day you start.

[1] "What's really propping up the economy" *BusinessWeek*, September 25, 2006.

Planning a Program of Study

Degrees in healthcare management are available at bachelor's, master's and doctoral level. Most bachelor's programs offer students three options: 1) general management; 2) specialist training in a specific discipline such as financial management or 3) focus on a specific segment of the industry such as ambulatory care or long-term care. AUPHA conducts a certification process for undergraduate programs in healthcare management.

An undergraduate degree in healthcare management can serve students in a variety of ways. For the student confident in wanting an administrative career in a sector of the healthcare industry, the undergraduate program can provide the basic knowledge, skills and applied studies needed for certain entry-level positions. It can also be the springboard to a graduate program for those seeking higher-level positions in healthcare management. For the clinician, the undergraduate program can provide a course of study in healthcare management and prepare them for leadership positions within their clinical specialty. For the student who wants to be a clinician, the undergraduate program can provide the foundation in learning they need to go on to their chosen area. Lastly, the undergraduate degree can also serve as a general management program which can be applied to other service industries.

A B.S. or B.A. degree — in any field of study — is the primary prerequisite for admission to a graduate program. In the past most students chose the traditional route of a master's degree in health administration or public health. Today, however, students are investigating other options, including degrees in business with course concentration in health services management. Some schools offer a joint degree — a master's degree in both business administration and public health, or in both healthcare management and law, for example. Graduate programs generally last two years and lead to a master's degree. They include coursework in healthcare policy and law, marketing, organizational behavior, healthcare financing, human resources, and other healthcare management topics. This program may also include a supervised internship, residency, or fellowship.

The Commission on Accreditation of Healthcare Management Education (CAHME) accredits master's level programs that prepare healthcare administrators according to established criteria. Only CAHME-accredited graduate programs may become full graduate members of AUPHA.

Executive education and continuing education programs in healthcare management are available for those currently employed in the field who want to broaden their knowledge and improve their skill base.

A doctoral degree in healthcare management, administration, research and policy, which is offered by many AUPHA member universities, or a doctoral degree in a related discipline — economics, political science, accounting, etc. — is the highest academic credential that can be earned.

What is certification and accreditation of a healthcare management program?

Graduate Accreditation

The CAHME accreditation is designed to foster high-quality, professional healthcare management education. "Healthcare Management" is an inclusive term describing skills and competencies utilized by individuals working to support and improve the delivery of health services. The definition involves many market segments, including (but not limited to) acute and non-acute providers, medical practices, community health organizations, insurers, pharmaceutical and equipment suppliers, professional societies and trade associations, consultants, health policy organizations, and the academic community.

Students can identify graduate management education programs that meet their chosen profession's standards by connecting to the CAHME website (www.cahme.org) and reviewing the requirements and curriculum of the CAHME accredited programs. The accrediting process assures students that the programs meet rigorous academic standards that prepare them for meaningful professional careers. All education programs seeking accreditation by CAHME, regardless of the setting for the graduate program, are evaluated by CAHME Criteria for Accreditation.

Undergraduate Certification

Hundreds of schools across the U.S. advertise undergraduate programs in health administration, healthcare management or health policy. The academic offerings for these programs range from a couple of electives in the subject added to a business degree on one end of the spectrum to a Bachelor of Health Administration with required field experience on the other. Within this wide range of available options, how does a program set itself apart from the others in terms of overall quality? How can prospective students gain the confidence and assurance that the academic program they choose is of the highest quality and relevant in today's healthcare industry? How can employers have confidence in the quality and competence of program graduates? All of this can be accomplished by turning to an AUPHA Certified Undergraduate Program.

For undergraduate healthcare administration programs, AUPHA has established a peer review process for those programs willing to undergo the rigors of external review in the interest of program excellence. Successful completion of the panel review process leads to Certification by AUPHA and attainment of Full Certified membership status. For a full list of Certified undergraduate programs go to www.aupha.org/custom/directory/programs.cfm?progtype=Undergraduate

The Admissions Process

The admissions process varies from school to school, largely dependent on whether school is house in a school of business, a school of public health or a school of nursing, among others. In order for the specific requirements of specific programs, potential students can refer to the AUPHA Healthcare Management Education Directory of programs, available in print or online at www.aupha.org > Publications > Directory of Healthcare Management Education

Helpful Links:

- Association of University Programs in Health Administration (www.aupha.org)
- American College of Health Care Administrators (www.achca.org)
- American College of Healthcare Executives (www.ache.org)
- ACHE's Healthcare Management Careers (www.healthmanagementcareers.org)
- American College of Medical Practice Executives (www.mgma.com/acmpe/index.cfm)
- American College of Physician Executives (www.acpe.org)
- American Organization of Nurse Executives (www.aone.org)
- Canadian College of Health Services Executives (www.cchse.org)
- ExploreHealthCareers.org (www.explorehealthcareers.org)
- Healthcare Financial Management Association (www.hfma.org)
- Healthcare Information and Management Systems Society (www.himss.org)
- Medical Group Management Association (www.mgma.com)
- National Association of Advisors to the Health Professions (www.naahp.org)
- National Association of Health Services Executives (www.nahse.org)
- U.S. Department of Labor, Medical and Health Services Manager (www.bls.gov/oco/ocos014.htm)
- Health Resources and Services Administration (bhpr.hrsa.gov/kidscareers)
- "Your Career as a Healthcare Executive" (ACHE) (www.ache.org/carsvcs/ycareer.cfm)

For additional information on a career in healthcare management, contact the Association of University Programs in Health Administration (AUPHA) at aupha@aupha.org or (703) 894-0940.

NATUROPATHIC MEDICINE (N.D.)

General Description of the Profession

Naturopathic medicine blends centuries-old, natural, non-toxic therapies with current advances in the study of health and human systems, covering all aspects of family health from prenatal to geriatric care.

Naturopathic medicine concentrates on whole-patient wellness. The medicine is tailored to the individual patient and emphasizes prevention and self-care. The philosophy of naturopathic medicine is rooted in finding the underlying cause of the patient's condition rather than focusing solely on symptomatic treatment. Naturopathic doctors (N.D.s) serve as primary care providers, an area of great current and future demand. As such, N.D.s cooperate with all other branches of medical science to refer patients to other practitioners and specialists for diagnosis or treatment when appropriate. Patient conditions most commonly treated by naturopathic doctors include fatigue, menstruation and hormonal issues, allergies, depression/insomnia, thyroid problems, weight/appetite, cholesterol, gastrointestinal disorders, headaches/migraines, blood pressure issues, diabetes and fibromyalgia. Naturopathic doctors sit for national board examinations and are licensed practitioners.

The major distinction between the N.D. and M.D. is that the N.D. is trained to approach diagnosis and treatment from a "holistic" perspective, treating the whole person rather than simply treating the symptoms. Secondly, the N.D. receives specialized training in natural therapies such as botanical medicine and nutrition, in addition to the core medical training common to all licensed doctors.

With a sound diagnostic biomedical science background, Western history and physical examination, laboratory testing and diagnostic imaging, naturopathic doctors treat patients with a wide variety of modalities, including:

- Nutrition
- Botanical Medicine
- Physical Medicine
- Homeopathy
- Lifestyle Counseling
- Hydrotherapy
- Pharmacology
- Minor Office Procedures
- Acupuncture and Oriental Medicine*
  *Only in scope of practice in a few states.

As evidenced by the numbers of patients seeking their care, naturopathic doctors find themselves serving a growing patient population:

- More than 80 million Americans turn to complementary and alternative medicine (CAM) every year.

- Up from 42 percent a decade ago, 48 percent of American adults used at least one alternative or complementary therapy in year 2004.[5]

- The majority of adults (68 percent) have used at least one kind of CAM therapy in their lifetime.

- At least 1/3 of cancer patients turn to a CAM therapy, most commonly in combination with allopathic treatment.

Background of the Naturopathic Profession

Established as a profession at the end of the nineteenth century, naturopathic medicine came into its own in the United States in the early 1900s. In their early practices, naturopathic doctors made use of diet, exercise, hydrotherapy, osseous and soft tissue manipulation, clinical nutrition, and botanical and homeopathic medicines, drawing on traditional healing practices that have evolved over hundreds of years.

Mid-century, with the promise of new miracle cures from pharmaceutical drugs such as antibiotics and the growth of the "high tech" and pharmaceutically-based system of conventional medicine, the widespread use of holistic therapies began to decline. A resurgence then began in the 1970s and has continued throughout the past decade, with 68 percent of the U.S. population now utilizing some form of complementary and alternative medicine, including naturopathic medicine.

Patients pursue naturopathic medicine to help address the complex health problems which have become so prevalent today. Naturopathic doctors offer natural health care that is minimally invasive and non-toxic, is based on prevention and promotion of therapeutic life changes, and takes into account the needs of the whole person. The naturopathic doctor considers the physical, emotional, social and spiritual factors when establishing a comprehensive diagnosis and individualized treatment of each patient. By establishing healthy lifestyles and tapping into what Hippocrates called the healing power of nature, naturopathic doctors help patients return to and maintain the state of equilibrium known as health.

The Naturopathic Paradigm

Within naturopathic medicine, you will discover a dynamic philosophy and a distinct system of healing, both founded in a deep respect for the body's intrinsic healing capacity. Effective traditional therapies form the foundation of naturopathic treatment. While drawing on the tools of modern science and careful collaboration with other health care professions, naturopathic doctors are able to offer their patients safe, effective and holistic solutions for health and wellness.

Primary Care

As a naturopathic doctor, you will become a primary care provider who is accomplished in looking beyond symptoms to the root causes of disease. You can expect to:

- Offer a range of care, from pediatric to geriatric.
- Take the time to build relationships with patients.
- Educate, guide and empower patients to take responsibility for their own health.

Naturopathic doctors see their role in health care as complementary as well as primary, so they work cooperatively with other health professionals, referring and co-managing patients appropriately.

Naturopathic Medical Principles

Six fundamental principles guide every aspect of the naturopathic doctor's orientation to health and wellness:

First Do No Harm
Utilize the most natural, least invasive and least toxic therapies.

Identify and Treat the Causes
Look beyond symptoms to address the underlying cause of illness.

Prevention
Focus on promoting health, wellness and disease prevention.

Treat the Whole Person
View the body as an integrated whole in all its physical, emotional and spiritual dimensions.

Doctor as Teacher
Educate patients in the steps to achieving and maintaining health.

The Healing Power of Nature
Trust in the body's inherent wisdom to heal itself.

The Decision to Pursue Naturopathic Medicine

You may have heard of naturopathic medicine but do not yet understand the profession in sufficient detail to make a well informed career choice. As an N.D. school applicant, you should make an effort early in your undergraduate years to enhance your knowledge and understanding of the field. The best way to begin exploring naturopathic medicine is to speak with a licensed naturopathic doctor, through interviewing or shadowing in his or her practice. For more information on finding an N.D. near you, visit the American Association of Naturopathic Physicians (AANP) website www.naturopathic.org.

Because of the exploding interest in natural health care, there are more career opportunities in natural medicine than ever before. Graduates of naturopathic programs are establishing thriving practices, with many choosing multi-faceted careers. They are working as **primary care doctors** in private practice and in integrative clinics. They are working as **research scientists** and **faculty members** in both alternative and conventional medical institutions. And they're filling positions as:

- Public health administrators
- Research and development scientists in the natural products industry
- Consultants to industry, insurance companies, public service, political and other organizations
- Wellness educators
- Practitioners in medispas in the U.S. and abroad

The broad scope and flexibility of natural medicine allows naturopathic doctors to create careers and lifestyles suited to their personality, their goals, their values and dreams.

Outlook for the Future

The practice of naturopathic medicine offers a mutually beneficial synergy of both patients and providers. The number of N.D.s practicing has tripled over the past 10 years, no doubt in response to the growing patient interest. As the field grows, the naturopathic profession continues to spark the interest of those dissatisfied with conventional medicine, both patients and doctors alike.

As a result, the job market for N.D. graduates continues to expand, with multi-disciplinary practices including M.D.s and D.O.s hiring new grads as associates. Naturopathic doctors are also working on Indian reservations, in community health centers and in specialty fields such as diabetes, allergies, cancer, pediatrics and women's health. The emerging field of spa medicine is also beginning to hire N.D.s at resorts, on cruise ships and in planned communities. Efforts to license the practice of naturopathic medicine are currently underway in several populous states, potentially opening up additional opportunities for patients to access naturopathic medicine.

Planning a Program of Study

General Information

Naturopathic medicine students learn to treat a wide range of family health issues, to practice prevention and to promote wellness. Students of naturopathic medicine use the Western medical sciences as a foundation on which to build a thorough knowledge of holistic, non-toxic therapies. Through their coursework and clinical experience, they develop skills in diagnosis, disease prevention and wellness optimization.

During the first two years of study, the N.D. curriculum focuses on basic and clinical sciences, covering biochemistry, human physiology, histology, anatomy, macro and microbiology, immunology, human pathology, neuroscience and pharmacology.

The final two years offer comprehensive clinical training in the holistic and non-toxic approaches to disease treatment and prevention that distinguish naturopathic medicine. In their supervised, hands-on experience with patients, students learn to scientifically apply clinical nutrition, homeopathic medicine, botanical medicine, physical medicine, psychology, acupuncture, pharmacology and counseling (to encourage patients to make therapeutic lifestyle changes in support of their personal health).

Naturopathic medical schools develop healers with knowledge, discrimination and sensitivity. The demands on the student are great, but so also are the rewards. Learning within such a healing environment is challenging, inspiring and sustaining.

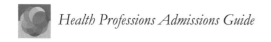
Choice of Undergraduate Major

Naturopathic medical colleges look for incoming students who demonstrate proficiency in the sciences and pursue a well-rounded curriculum. Most health professions advisors agree that you should select a major based upon your interests and aptitudes; you will therefore be more likely to enjoy your courses and to succeed in your chosen profession. Most of the N.D. programs require a base of undergraduate science courses that include physics, biology, and general and organic chemistry. Math and psychology courses may also be specified. Check with each school you are considering in order to ensure that all prerequisite requirements are met in advance.

In addition to the required coursework, other science courses to strengthen your background and to better prepare you for a naturopathic course of study include: anatomy, physiology, biochemistry, botany and developmental psychology. The Admissions Process

Background

Candidates should begin planning one to two years in advance. Submission of your application can begin as early as one year before your planned year of entry. Even though the "deadlines" for application are later than this, it is to your advantage to begin the application process as early as possible. All naturopathic medical colleges operate on a rolling admissions basis, so decisions are made throughout the application cycle.

Factors Evaluated by Admission Committees

In evaluating candidates for naturopathic medical programs, admissions counselors look for students who want to be challenged academically yet feel comfortable relying on their own intuition and creativity. They look for high-level critical thinkers who are flexible enough to deal with the challenge of formulating personalized treatment plans.

Applicants must demonstrate that they possess the internal qualities essential to becoming naturopathic doctors, including excellent communication skills, concern for others, integrity, curiosity, motivation and a strong belief in the philosophy and efficacy of naturopathic medicine. An aptitude for the sciences is important, as is overall intelligence. Prospective students must also demonstrate appropriate observational and interpersonal skills, motor function, intellectual-conceptual abilities, integrative and quantitative abilities, communication skills, and behavioral, emotional and social maturity.

1. **Academic Record**
   Entrance into an accredited naturopathic medical school requires extensive pre-medical course work and a bachelor's degree. Once you are enrolled, a naturopathic medical education promises a rigorous four-year curriculum, requiring in its first two years the same basic and clinical sciences required at allopathic medical schools. Some naturopathic medical schools do require more credit hours of basic science coursework than their allopathic counterparts.

   Admission committees at naturopathic medical schools are interested in admitting students who are well suited to becoming naturopathic doctors and have the academic ability to complete the program. Schools typically looks for candidates with a strong academic record, extracurricular activities, a commitment to volunteer work and exposure to the naturopathic medical profession.

2. **The Standardized Test (MCAT)**
   At this time, none of the naturopathic medical schools require their applicants to sit for the MCAT. However, many applicants do submit official scores with their application for admission.

3. **The Letters of Recommendation**

Most naturopathic medical colleges require a minimum of two letters of recommendation. Letters may be required from one or all of the following references: a faculty member or a previous instructor, a current or previous employer, and a naturopathic doctor or other licensed health care provider. Individual schools may have variations from this, so be sure to review the application materials from each school for directions as to the number and type of letters required.

4. **The Interview**

All naturopathic medical colleges require an in-person interview before admitting an applicant. The interview is an opportunity to demonstrate your knowledge and commitment to the field of naturopathic medicine. It also makes a good opportunity to continue exploring and learning more about the campuses of the schools to which you are applying.

5. **Extracurricular Activities and Work Experience**

As part of the application process, you will be asked to identify any and all extracurricular activities such as volunteer work, professional experience and community work.

6. **Age**

While most applicants fall within the 21 to 30 age range, applicants of all ages are considered by naturopathic medical schools, and you'll find students of all ages enrolled in the program.

The Application

1. **When and Where to Apply**

The application cycle begins on September 1. The schools are on a rolling admissions basis, and some offer "early decision" programs. By applying early, your materials will be processed in a more timely manner. Application deadline dates are established by each college, and therefore differ slightly among the schools.

2. **The Centralized Application Service**

At this time the naturopathic medical colleges do not utilize a centralized application service for applications. A standard application for admission should be obtained from and submitted directly to the naturopathic college to which you are applying.

Acceptance

1. **What You Can Expect from the Naturopathic Medical Colleges**

Most naturopathic medical colleges practice "rolling admissions"; some students are accepted before all applications have been processed or even received. Most naturopathic colleges will inform you of their admission decision within a few weeks after you are interviewed.

2. **What the Naturopathic Medical Colleges Expect from You**

Most letters of acceptance will specify a time period for you to accept the admission offer extended to you. At this time you will also be asked to place a tuition deposit (the amount varies with each college) to secure your seat in the class. If you choose to decline the offer it is helpful to the school and to other applicants to do so promptly.

Schools and Colleges of Naturopathic Medicine

The supporting organization for the naturopathic medical colleges in North America is the Association of Accredited Naturopathic Medical Colleges (AANMC). The association works to continually improve and maintain the quality of education among its member schools, and to enhance their visibility among prospective medical students.

Each of the naturopathic medicine programs of the AANMC member schools have been accredited (or are candidates for accreditation) by the Council on Naturopathic Medical Education (CNME), the recognized accreditor for naturopathic medical programs in North America.

The AANMC offers six affiliated North American ND schools to choose from – four in the U.S. and two in Canada. A complete listing of schools can be found at www.aanmc.org.

Resources

1. Association of Accredited Naturopathic Medical Colleges (AANMC), 4435 Wisconsin Avenue NW, Suite 403, Washington, DC 20016; www.aanmc.org.

    AANMC is the organization that works to advance the naturopathic medical profession by actively supporting the academic efforts of accredited and recognized schools of naturopathic medicine. A variety of links, resources, FAQ, and literature about the field of naturopathic medicine is available from the AANMC. Ask for a free copy of *Explore Naturopathic Medicine*. This can also be viewed online at www.aanmc.org.

    AANMC's website addresses many important issues in the field of naturopathic medicine, including definitions of the philosophy, the scope of practice, licensure and practice information. A description of each individual naturopathic medical college is also provided, along with contact information. You'll also find brief educational videos about the naturopathic medical colleges, as well as a subscription-based e-newsletter.

2. American Association of Naturopathic Physicians (AANP), 4435 Wisconsin Avenue NW, Suite 403, Washington DC 20016; 866/538-2267; www.naturopathic.org.

    The American Association of Naturopathic Physicians (AANP) is the national professional society representing licensed or licensable naturopathic doctors who are graduates of four-year, residential professional programs. The association's membership consists of more than 2,000 student, doctor, supporting and corporate members who collectively strive to expand access to naturopathic medicine nationwide.

4. Canadian Association of Naturopathic Doctors (CAND), 1255 Sheppard Ave. E., Toronto, Ontario, Canada M2K 1E2. 416/496-8633 www.naturopathicassoc.ca

    The Canadian Association of Naturopathic Doctors is the national professional society representing licensed or licensable naturopathic doctors in Canada.

3. Council on Naturopathic Medical Education (CNME), P.O. Box 178, Great Barrington, MA 01230; 413/528-8877; www.cnme.org.

    Founded in 1978, CNME is accepted as the programmatic accrediting agency for naturopathic medical education by the four-year naturopathic colleges and programs in the United States and Canada, by the American and Canadian national naturopathic professional associations, and by NABNE. CNME advocates high standards in naturopathic education, and its grant of accreditation to a program indicates that prospective students and the public may have confidence in the educational quality of the program. The U.S. Secretary of Education recognizes CNME as the national accrediting agency for programs leading to the doctor of naturopathic medicine (N.D. or N.M.D.) or doctor of naturopathy (N.D.) degree.

4. North American Board of Naturopathic Examiners (NABNE), 9220 S.W. Barbur Boulevard, Suite 19 #321, Portland, OR 97219-5434; 503/778-7990; www.nabne.org.

    NABNE administers and qualifies applicants to take the Naturopathic Physicians Licensing Examination (NPLEX) and also serves as an unbiased repository of exam scores, sending transcripts to licensing/regulatory authorities.

5. *The New York Times*, "Being a Patient" series, by Benedict Carey, February 2006.

NURSING (R.N., B.S.N., M.S.N.)

General Description

Nursing is the nation's largest health care profession with more than 2.9 million registered nurses nationwide. Despite its large size, many more nurses are needed into the foreseeable future to meet the growing demand for nursing care. As you plan or consider a career as a registered nurse, you should know these facts:

- The U.S. Bureau of Labor Statistics projects that employment for registered nurses will grow faster than most other occupations through 2016.

- Nursing students comprise more than half of all health professions students.

- Nurses comprise the largest single component of hospital staff, are the primary providers of hospital patient care, and deliver most of the nation's long-term care.

- Most health care services involve some form of care by nurses. Although 56.2 percent of all employed RNs work in hospitals, many are employed in a wide range of other settings, including private practices, public health agencies, primary care clinics, home health care, outpatient surgicenters, health maintenance organizations, nursing school-operated nursing centers, insurance and managed care companies, nursing homes, schools, mental health agencies, hospices, the military, and industry. Other nurses work in careers as college and university educators preparing future nurses or as scientists developing advances in many areas of health care and health promotion.

- Though often working collaboratively, nurses do not simply "assist" physicians and other healthcare providers. Instead, they practice independently within their own defined scope of practice. Nursing roles range from direct patient care to case management, establishing nursing practice standards, developing quality assurance procedures, and directing complex nursing care systems.

- With more than four times as many RNs in the United States as physicians, nurses deliver an extended array of healthcare services, including primary and preventive care by advanced, independent nurse practitioners in such clinical areas as pediatrics, family health, women's health, and gerontological care. Nursing's scope also includes care by clinical nurse specialists, certified nurse-midwives and nurse anesthetists, as well as care in cardiac, oncology, neonatal, neurological, and obstetric/gynecological nursing and other advanced clinical specialties.

- The primary pathway to professional nursing, as compared to technical-level practice, is the four-year Bachelor of Science degree in nursing (BSN). Registered nurses are prepared either through a four-year baccalaureate program; a two- to three-year associate degree in nursing program; or a three-year hospital diploma program. Graduates of all three programs take the same state licensing exam, the NCLEX-RN. (The number of diploma programs has declined steadily — to less than 10 percent of all basic RN education programs — as nursing education has shifted from hospital-operated instruction into the college and university system.)

To meet the more complex demands of today's health care environment, the National Advisory Council on Nurse Education and Practice has recommended that at least two-thirds of the basic nurse workforce hold baccalaureate or higher degrees in nursing by 2010. Aware of the need, RNs are seeking the BSN degree in increasing numbers. In 1980, almost 55 percent of employed registered nurses held a hospital diploma as their highest educational credential, 22 percent held the bachelor's degree, and 18 percent an associate degree. By 2004, a diploma was the highest educational credential for only 17.5 percent of RNs, while the number with bachelor's degrees as their highest education had climbed to 34.2 percent, with 33.7 percent holding an associate degree and 13.0 percent holding graduate degrees as their top academic preparation. In 2007, 14,946 RNs with diplomas or associate degrees graduated from BSN programs.

In addition, the American Association of Colleges of Nursing (AACN), the American Organization of Nurse Executives, the American Nurses Association and other leading authorities all recognize that the level of education makes a difference in nursing practice. The federal Health Resources and Services Administration is calling for baccalaureate preparation for at least two-thirds of the nursing workforce, due to evidence that clearly shows that higher levels of nursing education are linked with lower patient mortality rates, fewer errors, and greater job satisfaction among RNs. In addition, nurse executives, federal agencies, the military, leading nursing organizations, health care foundations, magnet hospitals, and minority nurse advocacy groups understand the unique value that baccalaureate-prepared nurses bring to the practice setting and their contribution to quality nursing care.

Additional ways of obtaining a BSN besides the traditional 4-year route include:
- Accelerated programs for adults with baccalaureate or graduate degrees in other fields (see below)
- RN to BSN degree completion programs for those with an associate degree or diploma in nursing. Many of these programs are offered online.
- Baccalaureate nursing programs offered at community colleges.

Rise of Accelerated Nursing Programs

Shifts in the economy and the desire of many adults to make a difference in their work have increased interest in the nursing profession among "second-degree" students. For those with a prior degree, accelerated baccalaureate programs offer the quickest route to becoming a registered nurse with programs generally running 12-18 months long. Generic master's degrees, also accelerated in nature and geared to non-nursing graduates, generally take three years to finish. Students in these programs usually complete baccalaureate-level nursing courses in the first year followed by two years of graduate study.

Graduates of accelerated programs are prized by nurse employers who value the many layers of skill and education these graduates bring to the workplace. Employers report that these graduates are more mature, possess strong clinical skills, and are quick studies on the job. Many practice settings are partnering with schools and offering tuition repayment to graduates as a mechanism to recruit highly qualified nurses.

In 2007, 205 accelerated BSN and 55 accelerated master's degree programs were offered at nursing schools nationwide. For more information on the accelerating nursing program and for a listing of schools offering this degree, go to www.aacn.nche.edu/Media/FactSheets/AcceleratedProg.htm.

Graduate Nursing Preparation

Though there is a great demand for nurses to provide direct care at the bedside, nurses with graduate preparation are also in high demand as advanced practice specialists, researchers, healthcare administrators, policy analysts, educators, and nurse executives. For students interested in pursuing graduate nursing education, examples of these programs include:

- Clinical Nurse Specialists
- Nurse Practitioner
- Nurse Midwife
- Nurse Anesthetist
- Clinical Nurse Leader
- Variety of Doctoral Studies (i.e. PhD, Doctorate of Nursing Practice or DNP)

Prepared typically in graduate programs, these advanced practice registered nurses (APRNs) include the following categories of clinicians:

- **Nurse Practitioners (NPs)** conduct physical exams; diagnose and treat common acute illnesses and injuries; provide immunizations; manage high blood pressure, diabetes, and other chronic problems; order and interpret X-rays and other lab tests; and counsel patients on adopting healthy lifestyles and health care options as a part of their clinical roles. In addition to practicing in clinics and hospitals in metropolitan areas, the nation's estimated 141,209 nurse practitioners also deliver care in rural sites, inner cities, and other locations not adequately served by physicians, as well as to other populations, such as children in schools and the elderly. Many NPs work in pediatrics, family health, women's health, and other specialties, and some have private practices. Nurse practitioners can prescribe medications in all states, while many states have given NPs authority to practice independently without physician collaboration or supervision.

- **Clinical Nurse Specialists (CNSs)** provide care in a range of specialty areas, such as cardiac, oncology, neonatal, and obstetric/gynecological nursing, as well as pediatrics, neurological nursing, and psychiatric/mental health. Working in hospitals and other clinical sites, CNSs provide acute care and mental health services, develop quality assurance procedures, and serve as educators and consultants. An estimated 72,000 clinical nurse specialists are currently in practice.

- **Certified Nurse-Midwives (CNMs)** provide prenatal and gynecological care to normal healthy women; deliver babies in hospitals, private homes, and birthing centers; and continue with follow-up postpartum care. In 2002, CNM deliveries accounted for 8.1 percent of all births in the U.S., up from 6.5 percent in 1996, according to the National Center for Health Statistics. There are approximately 13,700 CNMs nationwide.

- **Certified Registered Nurse Anesthetists (CRNAs)** administer more than 65 percent of all anesthetics given to patients each year, and are the sole anesthesia providers in approximately two-thirds of all rural hospitals in the U.S., according to the American Association of Nurse Anesthetists (AANA). Of the 24 million anesthetics given annually, about 20 percent are administered by CRNAs practicing independently and 80 percent by CRNAs in collaboration with physician anesthesiologists, says AANA. Working in the oldest of the advanced nursing specialties, CRNAs administer anesthesia for all types of surgery in settings ranging from operating rooms and dental offices to outpatient surgical centers. There are more than 32,600 CRNAs in practice nationwide.

Mounting studies show that the quality of APN care is comparable to MD's when they have the same level of authority, responsibilities, productivity, and administrative requirements (Mundinger, *JAMA, 2000; Medical Care Research and Review,* 2004). For example, inpatient surgical mortality is not affected by whether the anesthesia provider is a CRNA or an anesthesiologist (Pine, *AANA Journal,* 2003). Data from NP's working with the elderly show that they provide effective care to hospitalized geriatric patients, particularly older and sicker patients (Lambing, *Journal of the American Academy of Nurse Practitioners,* 2004). Physicians know and understand that they are limited in caring for so many sick patients. Michael E. Whitcomb, MD recently stated, "Since the supply of physicians will not be adequate to care for the increasing population of patients with chronic disease, academic medicine's leadership must place the needs of the patients in the forefront and work with the leadership of nursing to determine how best to provide the care those patients will need. It is simply unacceptable to have the needs of those patients go unmet." (*Academic Medicine,* 2006)

Though currently offered at the master's level, AACN member institutions voted to move the education level required for advance nursing specialist roles to the doctoral level by the year 2015. Doctoral preparation is the preferred level of education for nurse faculty, one of the greatest areas of need in the profession. Nurse educators play a central role in preparing new nurses and adapting curriculum in response to changing technology and professional practices.

The Decision to Pursue Nursing

Some of the most common reasons nurses state they pursued nursing include:

- **Competitive salaries:** New RNs can earn up to $55,000+ annually; advance practice registered nurses can command six-figure salaries.

- **Job security:** According to the American Hospital Association, three-quarters of all vacancies in hospitals are for RNs.

- **Career outlook is bright:** The Bureau of Labor Statistics has identified registered nursing as one of the top occupation in terms of job growth through the year 2016. There is an immediate need today for 116,000 nurses to fill vacancies in the nation's hospitals .Government analysts also project that more than 500,000 new RN positions will be created through 2016, which will account for two-fifths of all new jobs in the health care sector.

- **Endless opportunities and flexibility in workplace:** Nursing offers a wide array of professional practice opportunities in a variety of clinical settings. For example, though acute care facilities employ the highest number of nurses, home health care agencies, clinics, hospices, universities, armed forces, and large companies also employ nurses. Within these settings, nurses are educated to work with patients across the life span, from the neonate to the older adult. The choices in specialization are immense, including, pediatrics, critical care, psychiatry, dialysis, oncology, transplant, emergency room, community health, hospice/palliative care, geriatrics, among others. Nurses with advanced education also fill a variety of leadership roles including nursing faculty, administrator, researcher, policymaker, and independent practitioner.

- **No other healthcare team member spends more time at the bedside than the nurse.** The nurse is highly valued for his/her contribution to the care of patients, whether they are working in a clinic, in an acute-care facility, or out in the community as a visiting nurse. Because of their unique role in having a large amount of time with patients, their assessments are crucial to the interdisciplinary plan of care and patient safety.

Personal Attributes

Most successful nursing students possess a common set of attributes. These include:

- Strong science, math and communication skills
- Desire to advocate for patients and their families
- Desire to educate the community on health awareness and disease prevention
- Able to communicate with other members of the interdisciplinary team
- Skilled at coordinating care across many settings (i.e. acute care facility, homecare, long-term care, etc)
- Able to provide compassionate care for patients across the lifespan and their unique needs
- Desire to continue to learn, as practice constantly changes in regards to treatments, medications, etc.

Rewards of the Profession

The desire to help others is one of the primary rewards of being a nurse. No other healthcare professional spends more time at the bedside than the nurse. The profession offers a wide variety of educational opportunities. In addition, nurses have a diverse choice of clinical settings, such as clinics, acute care facilities, homecare, long-term care/skilled nursing facilities, hospice, military hospitals, etc. Opportunities to specialize in various subspecialties are appealing, as well. For example, nurses can work in neonatology, pediatrics, anesthesia, obstetrics, gynecology, endocrinology, oncology, cardiology, pulmonology, geriatrics, education, and research. Many nurse practitioners, clinical nurse specialists, and nurse midwives work autonomously.

Outlook for the Future

Federal figures project that if current trends continue, the shortage of RNs will continue to grow throughout the next 20 years. By 2025, more than 500,000 RN positions are expected to go unfilled nationwide, according to the latest data reported by leading workforce analysts Peter Buerhaus from Vanderbilt University. But already, in an expanding number of markets, hospitals and other employers are struggling to meet the rising demand for RN care and have stepped up recruitment.

Today's intensified hiring of RNs is being spurred by:
- the mounting health care needs of increasing numbers of elderly;
- a growing population of hospitalized patients who are older, more acutely ill, and in need of more skilled RNs per patient;
- the rapid expansion of front-line primary care to many sites throughout the community;
- technological advances requiring more highly skilled nursing care; and
- an aging RN workforce. The average age of working RNs in 2004 was 46.8 up from 40 in 1980. Moreover, only 8.1 percent of RNs were under age 30 in 2004, with high levels of retirements projected in the next 10 to 15 years.

As nursing and healthcare delivery expand, opportunities abound outside the hospital. Between 1996-2004, the number of registered nurses in community health settings, including home health care rose to 14.9 percent. An estimated 11.5 percent of RNs were practicing in outpatient settings in 2004, including health maintenance organizations and physician- and nurse-based practices, and 6.3 percent of RNs work in long-term care facilities.

With patient care growing more complex, ensuring a sufficient RN workforce isn't merely a matter of how many nurses are needed, but rather an issue of preparing an adequate number of nurses with the right *educational mix* to meet health care demands. The National Advisory Council on Nurse Education and Practice has urged that at least two-thirds of the basic nurse workforce hold baccalaureate or higher degrees in nursing by 2010. Currently, only 47.2 percent do.

Moreover, a 1995 report by the Pew Health Professions Commission called for a more concentrated production of nurses from bachelor's- and graduate-degree programs. Today's rising need for registered nurses does not appear to be a repeat of the widespread nursing shortage of a decade ago, when employers hired qualified entry-level RNs virtually regardless of their nursing degree preparation.

Rather, today's demand is different because:

- Employers are seeking nurses prepared at the bachelor's and graduate-degree levels who can deliver the higher complexity of care required across a variety of acute-care, primary-care, and community health settings, and to provide other needed services such as case management, health promotion, and disease prevention.

- Demand is particularly acute for nurses in key specialties, such as critical care; neonatal nursing; emergency, operating room, and labor and delivery units; and for advanced practice RNs such as nurse practitioners and clinical nurse specialists.

- Though hiring of RNs is accelerating in more cities, today's demand varies region by region, market by market, contrary to the pervasive nationwide shortfall of RNs in the late 1980s.

All projections forecast accelerating demand for nursing care and for nurses with expanded education and skills. Still, the demand for RNs varies by region and market. As a result, flexibility will be key for both entering and moving within the profession. Some graduates may need to pursue employment in different parts of their home states, in another state, or even in another region where hiring in certain clinical settings or specialties may be more plentiful.

Planning a Program of Study

Because there are many educational variations to becoming a nurse, visit the following website for planning a program of study: www.aacn.nche.edu/Education/nurse_ed/nep_index.htm.

In addition, baccalaureate nursing students must complete a variety of liberal arts studies, math and science courses (i.e. chemistry, anatomy and physiology, microbiology, etc) before entering nursing training. Students complete hours of clinical training in labs, hospitals, community settings, etc.

The Admissions Process

Each school of nursing has its own unique admission qualifications. However, with placements in nursing school being so very competitive, nursing schools can afford to choose exceptional students. Certain factors include:
- Excellent GPA
- Community service
- Letters of recommendation

Interested students should contact nursing schools as early as possible to determine program entry requirements, as they vary from school to school and competition for acceptance in nursing programs is very competitive.

Resources

1. American Association of Colleges of Nursing. (2008). Nursing Shortage Fact Sheet. Accessible online at www.aacn.nche.edu/Media/FactSheets/NursingShortage.htm.

2. Fang, D, Htut, A., Bednash GD. (2008) *2007-2008 Enrollment and Graduations in Baccalaureate and Graduate Programs in Nursing.* Washington, DC: American Association of Colleges of Nursing (AACN).

   - Career profiles in nursing
     - www.discovernursing.com
     - www.nursesource.org
     - www.nsna.org
   - Locating nursing programs
     - www.aacn.nche.edu
     - www.petersons.com
   - Financial aid for nursing students
     - www.aacn.nche.edu/Education/finaid.htm

Contact Person: Pam Malloy, MN, RN, OCN, American Association of Colleges of Nursing (AACN), pmalloy@aacn.nche.edu.

OCCUPATIONAL THERAPY (O.T.)

General Description

Occupational therapy is the art and science of helping people do the day-to-day activities that are important and meaningful to their health and well-being. It uses everyday activities as the means of helping people achieve independence and productive living. At the core of occupational therapy is the commitment to focus on the clients/patients as active agents seeking to accomplish their daily activities and roles in society.

Occupational therapists make it possible for people who face physical, cognitive, or mental health changes to participate more fully in their life roles at home and at school, at work, and at play. They are experts in helping patients use daily activities (occupations) to reach their full potential. They adapt the environment to maximize the patients' skills. By developing rapport with the patient and using creative problem-solving skills, they motivate patients and help them return to the roles that define them.

The types of services that occupational therapists provide include customized treatment programs to improve people's ability to perform daily activities; evaluation and treatment to develop or restore sensorimotor, cognitive, or psychosocial performance skills; comprehensive home and job site evaluations with adaptation recommendations to make them safe, conserve energy, enhance comfort, independence and productivity; adaptive equipment recommendations and usage training; and guidance to family members and caregivers.

A wide variety of people of all ages can benefit from occupational therapy services, including, for example, those with work-related injuries including lower back problems or repetitive stress injuries; arthritis, multiple sclerosis, or other chronic conditions; birth injuries, learning problems, or developmental disabilities; mental health or behavioral problems including Alzheimer's disease, schizophrenia, and post-traumatic stress; and limitations following a stroke or heart attack.

Occupational therapy practitioners work in a great variety of settings, including hospitals, nursing facilities and rehabilitation centers, home health agencies, clinics, schools and early intervention centers, industry, group homes and mental health facilities, academic programs (education and research), government agencies and many others. The clients they serve range in age from the very young (infants) to the very old.

Outlook for the Future

Currently, school systems, hospitals, and long-term care facilities are the primary work settings for a large number of occupational therapy practitioners. Other areas of practice are becoming increasingly important, and will become new specialties. They include training workers to use proper ergonomics on the job, helping people with low vision maintain their independence, making buildings and homes accessible, promoting health and wellness, and driving assessment and training for older adults and people with disabilities.

The job outlook for occupational therapy practitioners (occupational therapists and occupational therapy assistants) is excellent, and it is anticipated that the profession will continue to grow much faster than average. The US Department of Labor lists occupational therapy as one of the 30 fastest growing occupations through the year 2012 with a projected growth of 34%.

About 3/4ths of occupational therapy practitioners are employed full-time and 1/4th are working part-time. With increased world globalization, job opportunities are available not only nationally but also internationally. Reports of employment of 2004 graduates cite that within 8 weeks of graduation 96% of occupational therapists (OTs) and 88% of occupational therapy assistants (OTAs) are employed. According to the Bureau of Labor Statistics the median annual earnings for OTs is $60,470 and for OTAs is $42,060. Salaries vary according to the specific practice settings, geographic location, and levels of advanced skills and education.

All states require occupational therapy practitioners to have graduated from an accredited occupational therapy program including passing the entry level certification examination administered by the National Board for Certification in Occupational Therapy (NBCOT). They also must become licensed in the state where they plan to work. Entry into the profession can be either after completing an associate (occupational therapy assistant) or a post-baccalaureate (occupational therapist).

Planning a Program of Study

Occupational therapists (OT) currently earn a master's degree or doctorate degree from a university/college program. Professional programs typically require course work concentrating on the biological and behavioral sciences, including biology, psychology, and sociology. In addition to the coursework, students complete at least 6 months of supervised clinical internships in a variety of health care and community settings.

Common prerequisite requirements for entry in to an OT program may include (but are not limited to): biology, anatomy, physiology, psychology, sociology, human development, and statistics. The Graduate Record Exam (GRE) is an admission criterion as well as some (paid or unpaid) experience in working with people in a health or OT setting.

Applicants seeking a career in occupational therapy should possess strong interpersonal skills, an ability to work in teams, and a desire to help others. Additionally, being a creative problem-solver, a good listener, and a resourceful and compassionate person with an interest in health, science, and the arts are also desirable qualities.

Occupational therapy is a highly rewarding and personally satisfying profession. Entry into occupational therapy programs is competitive. Specific programs can be found through the American Occupational Therapy Association (AOTA).

Occupational therapy assistants (OTA) earn a 2-year associate degree from an occupational therapy assistant program. They will generally work under supervision of an occupational therapist.

Resources

The American Occupational Therapy Association
4720 Montgomery Lane
Bethesda, MD 20814-3425
(301) 652-2682
www.aota.org

US Department of Labor
Bureau of Labor Statistics
Occupational Outlook Handbook 2004-2005
www.bls.gov/oco

OPTOMETRY (O.D.)

General Description

Optometrists are the primary health care professionals for the eye. Optometrists examine, diagnose, treat, and manage diseases, injuries, and disorders of the visual system, the eye, and associated structures as well as identify related systemic conditions affecting the eye. Doctors of Optometry prescribe medications, low vision rehabilitation, vision therapy, spectacle lenses, contact lenses, and perform certain surgical procedures. Optometrists counsel their patients regarding surgical and non-surgical options that meet their visual needs related to their occupations, avocations, and lifestyle.

As an independent primary eye care provider, the optometrist is often the first to detect symptoms of eye disease including glaucoma and cataracts, as well as systemic diseases such as diabetes, hypertension and arteriosclerosis and, in some states, is able to treat eye diseases such as glaucoma. In each of these cases, s/he may refer the patient to the appropriate physician. The doctor of optometry also deals with vision problems that can be remedied through corrective refraction, either in the form of eyeglasses or contact lenses. Vision therapy for children helps them overcome learning problems due to vision deficiencies and provides them with the perception skills necessary for effective reading and studying. Another emerging area of optometric care is low vision rehabilitation, which provides sophisticated devices for individuals who formerly may have been classified as legally blind. The field of sports vision goes beyond vision screening to evaluate and teach vision skills that sharpen an individual's athletic performance. Optometrists are involved in determining safe vision standards in industry, and in determining who may safely drive an automobile.

At this time, most of the nation's practicing doctors of optometry are private optometric practitioners. These optometrists are in solo practice and the rest in associate partnerships and group practice. In an associate practice, a new practitioner practices with an established optometrist, thus avoiding capital investment costs to equip an office. The associate may take over or buy the office practice when the older optometrist retires. In group practice, two or more optometrists work in the same office, sharing costs and supplementing each other's vision specialties. Optometrists also practice in interdisciplinary group practices and may be members of the team of health care specialists. Optometrists also find employment in several branches of government service (they serve as commissioned officers in the Armed Forces), as well as in teaching and research.

The Decision to Pursue Optometry

Before contemplating devoting your life to optometry, you will want a clear picture of the profession. For a general overview of optometry, there is a DVD entitled, *The Eyes Have It*. Produced as an educational aid by the Association of Schools and Colleges of Optometry (ASCO), the DVD has been made available to health professions advisors around the country. This is an excellent introduction to the field of optometry; therefore, you will want to consult it early in your preparation. Also, refer to ASCO's website at www.opted.org for updated information.

In addition to a realistic view of the profession, you want to have a sense of your own aptitudes and inclinations, and be positive that your motivation for optometry is not only reality-based regarding the profession, but also appropriate for your personality and value system. One way to assure this is to visit and observe an optometrist at work; many practitioners welcome the opportunity to have potential students observe them and discuss their profession.

Personal Attributes

The desire to help others is one of the most important personality traits associated with the choice of a career in the health professions, and optometry is no exception. Skills for working with people are also important; the ability to communicate and to get along well with others is basic to the profession. You probably should enjoy working with your hands, since the optometrist must manipulate fine optical measuring devices and computer-controlled instruments. Since many optometrists are in independent practice, some business ability is desirable. In addition, if you are contemplating an optometric career you should have clear aptitude in the sciences and mathematics, since you will be studying a basic science curriculum during professional school.

Rewards of the Profession

Satisfaction from helping others is one of the primary rewards of being an optometrist. In addition to helping improve the quality of patients' lives, an optometrist is able to lead a satisfying personal life. The profession lends itself to very flexible working hours, and an optometrist's responsibilities do not normally include life-or-death decisions. Furthermore, forecasts for the profession indicate financial security in the present and opportunities in the future. Income is one of the rewards; the mean income for a self-employed optometrist in 2007 was $175,329. Finally, optometrists are accorded status in the community as providers of an essential health care service.

Outlook for the Future

The outlook for the future for optometrists is excellent. The American Optometric Association estimates that a ratio of one practicing optometrist to every 7,000 people would be a reasonable average for the United States. Few states currently meet this criterion, indicating a continuing need for more practitioners.

As people have come to expect improved eye care and as increasingly sophisticated technology has been developed to implement that care, the role of the optometrist is expanding. The growth of the geriatric population and the increasing vision problems that occur with age also point to an increased need for the optometrist. All of the trends mentioned above will probably continue to develop, and they are all undoubtedly responsible for the optimistic future employment prediction by the U.S. Department of Labor.

At the same time, it seems reasonable to assume that optometry, along with other health professions, will follow the direction that medicine has been moving. Affected by both business and government, the trend will likely be towards somewhat less entrepreneurship and more group practice, with a tendency for some practitioners to become employees in such entities as HMOs and other managed care settings.

Planning a Program of Study

General Information

Doctors of optometry receive four years of specialized professional education and clinical training at an accredited school or college of optometry after completion of their undergraduate prerequisites. There are nineteen accredited optometry schools in the United States. Information about all of these schools is included in the excellent handbook, *Schools and Colleges of Optometry Admission Requirements.* This is updated yearly and published by the Association of Schools and Colleges of Optometry (see Resources). The handbook is available on the ASCO website at www.opted.org. In addition, you will also want to consult the websites of the individual schools for more exact requirements.

Although the majority of all optometric students have a college degree, the minimum requirement for all optometry schools is completion of 90 semester units of college coursework. Specific admission requirements differ widely among the schools. One sensible strategy would be to prepare for an appropriate school with the most requirements, so that you will be eligible for the majority of schools with fewer required courses.

A list of courses the schools and colleges of optometry require of applicants follows. All science courses must be those designed for pre-professional students and must include laboratories. Brief survey courses in the sciences will not prepare you for optometry school.

Required Courses

Biology (all schools)	1 year
General Chemistry (all)	1 year
Organic Chemistry (all)	1 semester/1 year
Physics (all)	1 year
English (all)	1 year
College Algebra/Trigonometry/Calculus (all)	1 year
Psychology (most schools)	1 semester/1 year
Microbiology or bacteriology (most)	1 semester
Anatomy and Physiology (some)	1 year

Choice of Undergraduate Major

In addition to the basic science requirements, optometry schools emphasize preparation in mathematics and statistics, and most of them require at least one course in psychology. Optometric training involves optics and lens design. Optometry schools emphasize the necessity for applicants to be well versed in the sciences and to have a facility for dealing with people. Beyond requiring completion of their specific requirements and pursuit of a well-rounded curriculum, including the humanities and social sciences, the majority of schools do not express a preference for an undergraduate major. The schools that specify preferred majors list biology, psychology, or physical sciences.

If a specific major is not crucial to admission to optometry school, on what basis should you choose one? Most health professions advisors suggest that you select a major based on your interests and aptitudes, so that you will enjoy your courses and do well in them. Should you change your mind about optometry or be unable to gain admission to optometry school, a major should also provide an acceptable alternative career choice. Whatever your major, you need to be aware that the admission committee will evaluate the rigor of the program you elect along with the specific courses you undertake. Optometry schools teach you sciences at advanced levels and in heavy schedules. As an undergraduate, if you take only one science at a time, surrounded by liberal arts courses, you would not prove conclusively that you could handle the heavy science loads that are common during the first two years of optometry school. Two laboratory courses during each semester or quarter appear to be a good standard. However, you would be wise to discuss your situation with your health professions advisor.

The Admission Process

Background

For approximately two years, optometry students are taught mainly in the lecture format and in the laboratory, in a heavily scheduled block of courses in the basic health and visual sciences. How students perform in science courses in college predicts performance at this stage. This accounts for the fact that optometry schools emphasize the science grade point average and the course loads you took as an undergraduate.

Optometry students spend the next two years of optometry school studying diagnostic and treatment techniques in clinical settings. This clinical portion of the training calls for certain personal qualities, communication skills, and an educational background that will make you an effective practitioner. These are the character traits that are evaluated by your extracurricular activities, interaction with others, and communication skills exhibited in essays and during your interview.

Factors Evaluated by Admission Committees

An admission committee selects the entering class in each optometry school. The size as well as the composition of the committee varies from school to school, but it will normally be composed of ODs from the clinical faculty as well as PhDs from the basic science faculty. It may contain some third- or fourth-year optometry students. The composition of the committee can and probably will change from year to year. In general, optometry schools select students for their entering class who show evidence of strong intellectual ability, a good record of accomplishments, and personal traits that indicate the ability to communicate with and relate to patients.

Because admission committees strive for objectivity in making their decisions, they emphasize grades, scores on the Optometry Admission Test (the admission test which will be discussed below), and other factors that can be easily quantified. The four most important factors in determining whether or not you will be accepted to optometry school will usually be: (1) your academic record, (2) your scores on the OAT, (3) composite faculty evaluations, and (4) your personal interview. Other factors that will affect your acceptance are your understanding of optometry as a profession based on work experience, research, and/or discussions with doctors of optometry, and your extracurricular activities. Each of these will be discussed below.

1. **Academic Record**

   Most optometry school admission committees feel that the quality of work in the subjects taken to earn the baccalaureate degree may be the most important predictor of success in optometry school. The academic record includes the cumulative GPA, the science GPA (biology, chemistry, physics and mathematics), the subjects taken, the rigor of the program, and trends in performance. The latter consideration is important: a poor freshman year followed by subsequently better sophomore and junior years is preferable to a good freshman year followed by a declining performance. A good academic record is considered evidence of both high motivation and ability.

   Grades are not evaluated in a vacuum, but rather in context of your total time commitments. For example, part-time work or varsity athletics will be taken into account. However, the optometry school admission committees still need evidence of your ability to perform academically at an acceptable level.

2. **The Optometry Admission Testing Program (OAT)**

   All schools and colleges of optometry in the United States and Canada require the Optometry Admission Test (OAT). The OAT is a standardized examination designed to measure general academic ability and comprehension of scientific information. Courses helpful in preparation for the OAT include: one year Biology/Zoology, one year General College Chemistry, one year Organic Chemistry, and one year College Physics. The tests are comprised exclusively of multiple-choice test items presented in the English language.

The OAT is offered in a computerized format. Testing is available year round. Examinees are allowed to take the computerized format of the OAT an unlimited number of times but must wait at least 90 days between testing dates. Only scores from the four most recent attempts and the total number of attempts will be reported.

The test is just over one-half day in length and consists of four parts:

I. Survey of the Natural Sciences (biology, general chemistry, organic chemistry)
II. Reading Comprehension
III. Physics
IV. Quantitative Reasoning

The Optometry Admission Testing Program may include pretest questions in some test sections. Un-scored pretest questions are included on the test in order to ensure that these questions are appropriate before they are included among the scored items. If pretest questions are included in a test section, additional time will be allotted to that section of the test. Pretest questions are intermingled with the scored questions; therefore it is important to answer all questions.

Total Testing Time for the OAT

Test Sections	Time Limits
Tutorial	15 minutes
Survey of the Natural Sciences	90 minutes
Reading comprehension Test	50 minutes
Break (optional)	15 minutes
Physics Test	50 minutes
Quantitative Reasoning Test	45 minutes
Post Test Survey	10 minutes
Pre Testing	Up to 25 minutes

Total Time 275 to 300 minutes depending on the number of pretest questions.

The time limit is indicated on the computer screen for each section. The Survey of the Natural Sciences and the Reading Comprehension Test are administered first. The Physics Test and the Quantitative Reasoning Test are administered after an optional 15 minute rest break.

The Survey of the Natural Sciences is an achievement test. The content is limited to those areas covered by an entire first-year course in biology, general chemistry, and organic chemistry. The test contains a total of 100 items: 40 biology items, 30 general chemistry items and 30 organic chemistry items. The time limit of the test is 90 minutes. Although the three science sections are identified, it is important that the examinees pace themselves since separate sub scores will be given for each section.

The Reading Comprehension Test contains passages typical of the level of material encountered in the first year of optometry school. Each passage is followed by 10 to 17 items, which can be answered from a reading of the passage. One should not try to answer the questions until the passage is understood thoroughly. The time limit of the test is 50 minutes. Although these materials contain only one passage, the actual Reading Comprehension Test contains three passages and has a total of 40 items.

The Physics Test is also an achievement test. The content is limited to those areas covered in a two-semester physics course. The test contains a total of 40 items. The time limit of the test is 50 minutes.

The Quantitative Reasoning Test measures the examinee's ability to reason with numbers, to manipulate numerical relationships, and to deal intelligently with quantitative materials. The test contains 40 items. The time limit of the test is 45 minutes. Calculators are not permitted.

Test preparation materials are available on the OAT website (www.opted.org). These materials contain samples of the four tests used in the Optometry Admission Testing Program. They are available to assist examinees in discovering possible areas of weakness in comprehension of subjects covered on the test. Sample tests also enable examinees to become familiar with the types of materials included in the test, as well as the general format of the various parts of the test battery.

a. **Reviewing for the Test**

If you know that you have poor test-taking skills on standardized/multiple-choice tests, you will want to address this problem well before the year in that you are scheduled to take the OAT exam. Have your reading, studying, and test-taking skills checked, and you might even investigate the area of test anxiety if it seems relevant. In order to work out an effective test-taking strategy, refer to the section "Standardized Tests" in Chapter 2.

A thorough review of biology, chemistry, physics and math requires a significant amount of time. It is a good idea to set aside a specific block of time each day, and adhere to this schedule. Old notes and textbooks are a valuable resource; the material tested is at the introductory level. The Optometry Admission Testing electronic practice test can serve as your guide. It lists every topic for which you will be responsible.

Taking the practice test before you begin to review may help you to structure your review, as well as to gain familiarity with the test format. Your results on this test serve as a diagnostic aid and "benchmark." The test can be repeated after your review has been largely completed (perhaps three weeks before the test). You can then address any weaknesses that are still evident. Each of these tests should be taken at one sitting, with no interruptions, and with the time limits strictly observed, i.e., under conditions simulating those of the actual test. If you have been organized in your review, you can stop studying two or three days before the test.

You might also use the sample test conditions to practice the techniques outlined in chapter 2. While all of these techniques are mechanical and do not depend on actual knowledge of the subject matter (and will not replace that knowledge), they can be extremely helpful in improving your score on any standardized examination.

b. **Scores and Their Interpretation**

The raw scores (based on the number of correct answers, with no penalty for guessing) are treated statistically and become standard scores for the sake of reporting. The scaled scores are reported in a range from 200 to 400. While there are no "passing" or "failing" grades, the standard score of 300 signifies average performance on a national basis.

3. **Letters of Evaluation**

Letters of evaluation are discussed in more detail in chapter 2. Optometry schools admission committees generally prefer an individual letter to a composite or committee evaluation. Telling the professors whom you plan to ask for evaluations that you are a pre-optometry student will help them write a more informed evaluation. Do not take it for granted that letters are sent. Keep in close contact with your health professions advising office in collecting these important supporting documents so you can be sure that they are sent out in a timely manner.

Some schools ask for additional letters or "character references." The school usually specifies whether these letters should come from optometrists, employees, friends, or others; it is a good idea to follow those guidelines. One school, for example, requires a letter from an optometrist, whereas another suggests that you do not send one from an OD. Regardless of the kind and number of evaluations required, it is your responsibility to check to see not only that they are written, but also that they have been received and filed under your name at every optometry school where you have applied.

4. **The Interview**

Most optometry schools interview their prospective students. An interview invitation represents a significant step in the selection process. Other applicants have already been screened out on the basis of their academic record and non-academic characteristics.

Once again, the general discussion contained in earlier pages can serve as your guide. You need to be prepared to talk about yourself in the interview and to have some knowledge of the field of optometry. Also helpful is information regarding the school where you are interviewing, including its particular strengths, special programs in teaching, or other innovative programs for its students. The school's catalog is a good source of this information, as are videotapes that several of the schools supply. Check with your health professions advising office to see if there are any of these available at your school.

5. **Extracurricular Activities and Work Experience**

Optometry schools view extracurricular activities as positive signs that you can handle a rigorous curriculum and still participate in campus or community affairs. Commitment, leadership, service, responsibility, and the ability to interact effectively with others are among the qualities that the optometry school admission committees evaluate. The level and quality of your participation is more important than the number or diversity of your activities. These activities include community service, campus involvement, research involvement and outside jobs, as well as interests and hobbies. Contrary to popular myth, however, extensive involvement in extracurricular activities, no matter how meaningful, will not compensate for an academic performance that is below par. It may instead indicate to admission committees that you have poor judgment, skewed priorities, and/or inadequate time-management skills.

6. **Experience with Optometry**

Working in an optometric setting can give you an opportunity not only to gain valuable experience, but also to help you in your own decision to pursue optometry as a career. You will have an opportunity to observe trained professionals in action and may have a chance to perform simple tasks. You will find out whether the professional role looks interesting, challenging, varied or whether it is different from your preconceived ideas.

Whichever is the case, this type of experience is of value. It demonstrates to the admission committees that you have taken more than a casual look at optometry as your career choice.

7. **Research Experience**

Research has become a significant area in optometry; optometrists now serve as members of National Institutes of Health committees — the government facility responsible for the majority of health research in the United States. The field of optometry has also made contributions to national defense in the development of special sighting and night vision equipment. Several schools of optometry offer graduate degrees in physiological optics for optometrists who want to enter research and/or teaching. If you think you might be interested in pursuing research as an optometrist, it would be a good idea to involve yourself in a research effort. Even if you are not interested in pursuing research as a profession, understanding concepts such as the scientific method, statistical significance, and the experimental process, will enable you to evaluate the research of others.

8. **The Value of Work**

Jobs unrelated to optometry may give you experience that will be beneficial in helping you develop better management and interpersonal skills. Jobs that require considerable contact with the public, for example, will help to develop interaction modes that will be useful in patient care. Jobs that involve management of both work and personnel help develop responsibility and a mature attitude. If you cannot afford to volunteer and cannot find a paying job with an optometrist, try to use whatever position you find in a constructive manner to develop some of these interpersonal skills. Any business acumen you develop will be of value to you as an optometric professional.

The Application

1. **When and Where to Apply**
   The application process typically begins during the summer or early fall, one year before you expect to begin optometry school. Taking OAT one year before you wish to enter will give you a chance to repeat the test if your scores are low. Use the handbook, *Schools and Colleges of Optometry Admission Requirements* for a preliminary look at all schools. Considering your own state residency, grade range, and OAT scores will help eliminate those schools that appear to be unrealistic. Your health professions advisor may have suggestions concerning your choice of schools and may be able to tell you where students at your school have been successful in the past. An early application will generally benefit you, because most of the schools use "rolling admissions" (i.e., they do not wait for their deadline to pass before processing applications; instead, they evaluate and accept applicants as their files are completed).

In deciding where to apply to optometry school, one of the prime considerations is your state of residence. Because there are so few schools of optometry, many states do not have a school but contract with specific schools to accept their residents preferentially, provide for partial tuition remission or both. You should determine whether there are places at the schools of your choice for people from your home state and whether your state has a contract with those schools. For example, many southeastern states have contracts with the University of Alabama at Birmingham and Southern College of Optometry, while Southern California College of Optometry, Pacific University College of Optometry and University of California, Berkeley have contracts via the WICHE program in western states. Consult school bulletins and contact individual schools for more specific information regarding contract arrangements for residents of your state. Your health professions advising office will have additional literature, videotapes, and other resource materials available for help with this selection process.

Launching in 2009 for Academic Year 2010-2011 is OptomCAS, the Optometry Centralized Application Service sponsored by the Association of Schools and Colleges of Optometry (ASCO). Through this service you will be able to file one application and send it to multiple optometry programs. At this time, all nineteen schools of optometry plan to participate. For more information, please check out www.optomcas.org.

2. **Follow Up**
   After submitting all the required materials through OptomCAS, each school you have applied to will contact you directly if they need addition information. It is your responsibility to check with OptomCAS to make sure your application is complete.

Resources

1. *Optometry: A Career Guide.* This book contains the latest available information for students interested in applying to optometry schools in the United States. The latest edition should be consulted by students when deciding where to apply. Available by writing to the Association of Schools and Colleges of Optometry, 6110 Executive Blvd., Suite 420, Rockville, MD 20852; 301/231-5944; www.opted.org.

2. Optometry Admission Testing (OAT) Electronic Examinee Guide & Practice Test. www.opted.org.

3. Association of Schools and Colleges of Optometry website. This informative site has information on optometric education in general, as well as information on the schools and colleges: www.opted.org.

For a complete list of the 19 schools and colleges of optometry, visit www.opted.org.

OSTEOPATHIC MEDICINE (D. O.)

General Description

The philosophy and practice of osteopathic medicine developed in reaction to the frequently harmful medicine being practiced in the United States in the late 1800s. Osteopathic medicine is a uniquely American branch of medicine that has continued to evolve in the United States through the scientific method of discovery. Today, U.S. osteopathic physicians (who hold the Doctor of Osteopathic Medicine degree and are known as D.O.s) are fully licensed, patient-centered medical doctors. They have full medical practice rights throughout the United States and in 44 countries abroad.

The early days of osteopathic medicine were marked by a lack of professional communication between the new field and the long-established field of allopathic medicine (Doctor of Medicine, known as M.D.). However, most barriers between the two forms of medical practice have been removed or reduced, and there is full acceptance of osteopathic medicine by the public and by medical licensing boards in each of the 50 states. Residency programs are available to D.O. graduates under the auspices of either the American Osteopathic Association (AOA) or the American Medical Association (AMA)/Accreditation Council for Graduate Medical Education. The major distinction between the D.O. and M.D. today is that the D.O. receives additional specialized training in osteopathic principles and practices, including the diagnostic and treatment method known as osteopathic manipulative medicine and the profession's distinctive philosophical approaches to patient-centered care and treatment. Another distinction is that osteopathic medicine emphasizes primary care. Approximately 65 percent of all osteopathic physicians practice in one of the primary care areas of family practice, internal medicine, pediatrics, or obstetrics and gynecology.

Today, nearly one in five students at U.S. medical schools is training to be an osteopathic physician, and the numbers are increasing each year. The nation's approximately 55,000 fully licensed osteopathic physicians practice the entire scope of modern medicine, bringing a patient-centered, holistic, hands-on approach to diagnosing and treating illness and injury.

Osteopathic physicians can be found in virtually all types of medical practice across the United States, ranging from general practice in small towns to highly specialized practice in the country's largest cities. However, the emphasis the profession places upon primary care bodes well for the future. Medical policy-making organizations, including the U.S. Department of Health and Human Services, agree that primary care is the area of greatest medical need, now and in the foreseeable future.

The vast majority of osteopathic medical students spends four years in undergraduate school and receive a bachelor's degree prior to entering medical school. Osteopathic medical education consists of four years of professional education, generally organized as two years of basic science courses and two years of clinical training. Much of the clinical training is composed of "clinical clerkships," where the student spends time in a clinical setting under the supervision of licensed physicians in preceptor roles. Clerkships are a part of the osteopathic medical school program and are separate and distinct from internship and residencies, which occur after graduation. It is possible to complete clerkships in a variety of clinical settings throughout the United States.

After receiving the D.O. degree, graduates may serve a 12-month internship approved by the American Osteopathic Association. Completion of this internship allows the new D.O. to begin the general practice of medicine. Graduates, however, may apply for entry into specialty training in a variety of M.D. or D.O. residency programs that range in length from two to six additional years. Graduates may enter residency programs either directly on graduation from medical school or following a one-year osteopathic internship (in some cases depending on state licensing regulations).

Licensure of the D.O. is established in each state, District of Columbia or U.S. territory by a medical examining board that conducts the licensure examination. Typically, this board exam is similar to that required for licensure of M.D.s in that jurisdiction. To become licensed as an osteopathic physician, one must successfully complete the Comprehensive Osteopathic Medical Licensing Examination (COMLEX), Levels I, II (a 2-part exam) and III. This examination is administered by the National Board of Osteopathic Medical Examiners (NBOME). Osteopathic medical students also are eligible to take the United States Medical Licensure Examination (USMLE), which has historically been used if the student intends to pursue allopathic graduate training, although many allopathic graduate programs accept COMLEX exams. Many states have reciprocity agreements, allowing passage of the licensure examination for one state to meet the requirement in other states. Regardless of the method of examination in each jurisdiction, licensure in the United States carries with it the full range of practice rights and privileges.

The Decision to Pursue Osteopathic Medicine

You may have heard of osteopathic medicine but have not had the opportunity to encounter sufficient detail to fully understand and appreciate the profession. Many applicants come face-to-face with the profession only when they reach the point of applying to osteopathic medical school. You should make a serious effort early in your undergraduate years to enhance your knowledge and understanding of the field.

A good way to learn about osteopathic medicine is to talk with or observe one or more osteopathic physicians. Many D.O.s are happy to help prospective applicants learn about the field. Interaction with several D.O.s provides a good understanding of what the profession might offer.

Outlook for the Future

The future of osteopathic medicine appears bright as the field continues to become better known to the public. In addition, osteopathic (D.O.) and allopathic (M.D.) medicine continue to move closer together in modes of practice and philosophy. Increasingly, D.O.s and M.D.s are collaborators in joint practices or in hospital settings, but osteopathic medicine will continue to retain those aspects of training, modes of practice and philosophy that make it unique.

Planning a Program of Study

General Information

There are 25 U.S. osteopathic medical colleges, three of which have branch campuses. The past 20 years have seen dramatic growth in the number of osteopathic medical schools. Nearly half of the colleges have been established during that time. The colleges are geographically spread across the U.S. The schools feature a remarkable consistency of philosophy and commitment to osteopathic medicine.

Most osteopathic medical colleges require one academic year (two semesters or three quarters) of the following courses: biology, with laboratory; general chemistry, with laboratory; organic chemistry, with laboratory; general physics, with laboratory; and English Composition. Several specify one academic year of behavioral sciences.

The pre-professional course requirements for every U.S. osteopathic medical college are listed in *The Osteopathic Medical College Information Book* (CIB), which is updated annually and can be viewed online at www.aacom.org/resources/bookstore/cib/Pages/default.aspx. You should become familiar with this resource early in your pre-professional program and determine precise course requirements for the specific osteopathic medical colleges to which you plan to apply. The required science courses typically should be completed by the end of the junior year of your undergraduate program, if you plan to begin medical school directly after college. These courses also are needed to prepare you for the Medical College Admission Test (MCAT). You have only three years to prove yourself academically if you plan to enter osteopathic medical school after graduation. The admission committees generally will not see your senior year transcript (especially the spring semester or quarter) before they make admission decisions. You may, of course, have more than three years of academic work if you are a returning student who is changing fields, or if you are pursuing a nontraditional academic schedule. Consult your health professions advisor regarding nontraditional course and application scheduling.

Some osteopathic medical colleges recommend coursework in addition to the required courses. Regardless of whether a particular school recommends it, a course in biochemistry is excellent preparation for the first-year biochemistry course in osteopathic medical college. Other recommended courses may include genetics, histology, cell biology, embryology and comparative anatomy. On the other hand, osteopathic schools stress the importance of a well-rounded undergraduate curriculum. Most recommend courses in the behavioral sciences, social sciences, humanities and fine arts. Extracurricular activities, volunteer work and clinical exposure to medicine are also important.

Choice of Undergraduate Major

In what should I major? Students planning medical careers often have the misperception that they should major in "pre-medicine." Few colleges or universities offer such degrees, and even fewer health professions schools would suggest that you major in such a program. Osteopathic medical college admission committees look for students who demonstrate proficiency in the sciences and have pursued a well-rounded curriculum.

Most health professions advisors agree that you should select a major based upon your interests and aptitudes; you are more likely to enjoy your courses and do well in them. If you change your mind about going into medicine or are unable to gain admission to medical school, a major can also provide preparation for an alternative career. Professions such as podiatric medicine, dentistry, optometry, veterinary medicine, pharmacy, nursing, and other clinical health career choices all have similar prerequisites and preparation.

The Admissions Process

Background

The admissions process should become an integral part of your thinking about 18 to 24 months prior to the time you anticipate matriculating into osteopathic medical school. The submission of your application through the centralized online application service can begin as early as May of the year before the year of entry. AACOMAS online is available at aacomas.aacom.org. Even though the "deadlines" for application are later, it is to your advantage to begin the application process as early as possible. All osteopathic medical colleges operate on a rolling admissions basis, so decisions are made throughout the application cycle. Classes may be filled and/or interview spots may be taken long before application deadlines are reached. Your health professions advisor can help you plan your application strategy, and you are encouraged to contact him/her early in the process.

Factors Evaluated by Admission Committees

- **Academic Record**
  Admission committees at osteopathic medical schools are interested in admitting students who are well-suited to becoming osteopathic physicians and have the academic ability to complete the program. You must recognize that you are competing with other applicants for a position in the class. Thus, it is to your advantage to establish an excellent academic record, but not at the expense of breadth. Achieve a good balance between time and effort spent on your academic work and extracurricular experiences. Consult your health professions advisor for an evaluation of your academic record within the context of an osteopathic medical school application.

- **The Standardized Test (MCAT)**
  All osteopathic medical schools require the Medical College Admission Test (MCAT) to consider an applicant for admission. It is recommended that the MCAT be taken no later than summer of the calendar year prior to the year of planned medical school matriculation. This allows you time to assess your performance and retake the test if necessary. For a more detailed discussion of the MCAT, see the section under allopathic medicine in this chapter. While some osteopathic medical schools will accept MCAT scores from the January administration in the year of matriculation, most will accept these scores only as an additional score.

- **The Letters of Evaluation**
  Most osteopathic medical colleges require a minimum of three letters of evaluation. Often, one of these letters must be from an osteopathic physician. The other two should be from science faculty who have taught you. Schools often prefer a letter of evaluation from a health professions committee, which may be a composite of other letters in your file. Individual schools may have varying supplemental materials requirements, so be sure to examine each school's application procedures for directions as to the number and type of letters required.

Although not all osteopathic medical colleges require a letter of evaluation from an osteopathic physician, it is to your advantage to become acquainted with one or more D.O.s. Ask your health professions advisor if s/he could introduce you to a D.O. Many state osteopathic medical associations maintain lists of D.O.s who are willing to talk with prospective osteopathic medical students. Colleges of osteopathic medicine are also excellent resources and may be able to refer you to a D.O. in your area. To locate your state osteopathic medical association address, contact the American Osteopathic Association at 800/621-1773; www.osteopathic.org or contact the American Association of Colleges of Osteopathic Medicine (AACOM) at www.aacom.org.

- **The Interview**

  Most osteopathic medical colleges require a personal interview before admitting an applicant. The interview is an opportunity to demonstrate your knowledge and commitment to osteopathic medicine. It is also an opportunity to visit the school and determine that the school is "right" for you. The interview is an opportunity for both the applicant and the college to assess each other.

  It is essential that you become familiar with the profession and can honestly say "I want to be an osteopathic physician because…" If you have just recently become aware of the profession, a good decision can be made only after you have read extensively about the profession and talked with osteopathic physicians.

- **Extracurricular Activities and Work Experience**

  You are encouraged, to the extent allowed by your academic work, to gain some experience outside the classroom. This will give you a broader perspective and will help you put your academic work and long-range professional goals into perspective. Gaining exposure to the general field of medicine will help you gain knowledge about the field, what it will demand of you, what its rewards and shortcomings are, and what its future holds.

The Centralized Application Service

The centralized application service for osteopathic medical schools is online at aacomas.aacom.org. Although there are 25 osteopathic medical schools (and three branch campuses), only 24 participate in AACOMAS (The University of North Texas Health Sciences Center — TCOM uses TMDSAS). The initial application to these schools is the standardized application submitted directly to AACOMAS, a web-based application. After AACOMAS has processed your application, application data are sent to each osteopathic school you designate.

After initial review and screening by an osteopathic medical college, you may receive a supplemental application to be returned directly to the college. Supplemental applications ask you to provide information that is unique to your interest in and application to a particular school. A request for letters of evaluation usually accompanies the supplemental application. You may also receive an invitation to interview either along with the supplemental application request or after completing the supplemental application.

Acceptance

- **What You Can Expect from the Osteopathic Medical Colleges**

  Most osteopathic medical college admission committees practice "rolling admissions"; some students are accepted before all applications have been processed or even received. Most osteopathic schools will inform you of a decision (acceptance, alternate status, or denial) within a few weeks following your interview. If you find yourself on one or more alternate lists, most admission committees are willing to keep you informed of your status.

- **What the Osteopathic Medical Colleges Expect from You**

  Most letters of acceptance will specify a time by which you must respond to the offer. If you plan to decline the offer, it is helpful to the school and to other applicants to do so promptly. On the other hand, you may plan to accept the offer, or you may need more information before you can make a final decision. You may need time to evaluate the financial picture, including financial aid availability at the schools to which you have been accepted. You will be asked to place a deposit (the amount varies from college to college) to secure your seat in the class. If you hold a position in more than one osteopathic or allopathic medical school, it is your responsibility to withdraw at the earliest possible date from all but the one where you plan to matriculate.

You may be informed that you are on one or more alternate lists. Movement on such lists is active up to the day classes begin. If you are on one or more lists, you are advised to have alternative plans in mind so that you can make a quick decision should this become necessary. Be aware, however, that you are no longer considered to be on an alternate list once you have matriculated at a medical college. Once matriculated, however, courtesy dictates that you inform all schools.

AACOMAS maintains guidelines and protocols for the application process. These are updated and published annually in the *Osteopathic Medical College Information Book* (CIB) and online.

Special Programs

Even though an individual osteopathic medical school may not publicize a special program, if you have a desire to include a special component in your program, it is to your advantage to ask whether this will be possible. For example, you may want to delay your date of matriculation or to work on a graduate degree at the same time you are working toward your D.O. degree. Each of these situations (and possibly others) may not be publicized but may be available upon request.

- **Joint Degree Programs**
  Most of the 25 COMS offer a variety of joint degree programs. The listing for these programs is quite extensive and can be found in the CIB.

- **Early Decision Programs**
  Several of the colleges of osteopathic medicine have official Early Decision Programs (EDP). Colleges offering EDP programs are listed in the CIB. Contact each school's Admissions Office for additional information.

Resources

1. American Association of Colleges of Osteopathic Medicine (AACOM), 5550 Friendship Boulevard, Suite 310, Chevy Chase, MD 20815-7231; 301/968-4100; www.aacom.org.

2. AACOM is the organization that serves the nation's colleges of osteopathic medicine and their students. A wide variety of literature about the field of osteopathic medicine is available from AACOM. AACOM's website addresses many important issues, including a discussion of the similarities and differences between the D.O. and M.D.

   For a complete list of the 25 colleges of osteopathic medicine, visit www.aacom.org.

   American Association of Colleges of Osteopathic Medicine Application Service (AACOMAS), 5550 Friendship Boulevard, Suite 310, Chevy Chase, MD 20815-7231; 301/968-4190.

   The AACOMAS application is a web-based application that can be accessed at the AACOM website.

   American Osteopathic Association (AOA), 142 East Ontario Street, Chicago, IL 60611-3269; 312/202-8000 or 800/621-1773; www.osteopathic.org.

   This is the osteopathic physician professional organization.

References about osteopathic medicine include:

The DOs: Osteopathic Medicine in America by Norman Gevitz, PhD

Osteopathic Medicine: A Reformation in Progress by R. Michael Gallagher, DO, FACOFP and Frederick J. Humphrey, II, DO, FACN.

FIRE ON THE PRAIRIE: The Life and Times of Andrew Taylor Still, Founder of Osteopathic Medicine by Zachary Comeaux

PHARMACY (Pharm.D.)

General Description

Pharmacists are the health professionals who serve patients and other health professionals in assuring appropriate use of, and optimal therapeutic outcomes from, medications. In addition to the responsibility for professional interpretation and review of prescription orders, medication record screening and review, and the accurate dispensing of medications, pharmacists serve patients and the community by providing information and advice on health, providing medications and associated services, and by referring patients to other sources of help and care, such as physicians, when necessary.

Pharmacists must be fully acquainted with the physical and chemical properties of drugs and the way they behave in the human body. They must know how a particular drug will affect a human being, alter the course of a disease, and react in the presence of other drugs. Pharmacists must also know how a drug may react in laboratory tests of blood and other human tissues.

Pharmaceutical care encompasses the full range of pharmacists' skills, knowledge, and ability in providing medication services to patients. The principle goal of pharmaceutical care is to achieve positive intended outcomes from medication use to improve patients' quality of life. These outcomes include: (1) cure of a disease; (2) elimination or reduction of symptoms; (3) arresting or slowing a disease process; (4) prevention of disease; (5) diagnosis of disease; and (6) desired alterations in physiological processes, all with minimum risk to patients. Pharmacists are professionals committed to public service and to the achievement of this goal.

Pharmacists may also require proficiency in business matters, since they may purchase and sell hundreds of health-related items. In the hospital, pharmacists assist physicians in drug therapy decisions and may be responsible for the selection and purchase of all medicines used by the facility. In settings where hiring and supervision of personnel is required, pharmacists need personnel and fiscal management capabilities. One of the primary roles of the pharmacists is to serve as an educator in the proper use of drugs for both the public and health practitioners.

The Decision to Pursue Pharmacy

Pharmacists must have excellent interpersonal and communications skills. To perform each of the described activities well, pharmacists must read biological, medical and chemical literature as well as professional, corporate and pharmaceutical publications. Being a member of the profession of pharmacy requires commitment and dedication to life-long learning.

Pharmacists assume responsibility for human life. They are dedicated to providing conscientious and dependable services and should enjoy working with people. Meticulous regard for accuracy, orderliness, and cleanliness is essential. Pharmacists' ethics must be unquestionable. They are entrusted with the storage and distribution of dangerous and habit-forming pharmaceuticals and must be scrupulous in handling or dispensing all medications.

The number of women in the profession of pharmacy has been increasing steadily: 32% in 1991, 46% in 2000, and over 50% in 2007. The Bureau of Health Professions projects 64% of pharmacists will be female by 2020. There is currently a nationwide shortage of pharmacists. The shortage is largely due to increased demand for pharmacists' services, including those associated with both drug distribution and direct patient care. Employment is expected to be stable for the foreseeable future with growth centered in chain store expansion, in ambulatory care centers, and in nontraditional practice areas. According to the Bureau of Labor Statistics, half of all pharmacists made $ 100,480 a year in 2006. The lowest 10 percent made $ 73,010 and the highest 10 percent earned $ 126,410 a year. According to a 2008 survey by Drug Topics magazine, the median annual earning of pharmacists was $107,403 in 2007, $94,927 in 2006, as compared to $89,723 in 2004, $82,607 in 2002, $78,624 in 2000, and $64,980 in 1999.

Since pharmacists have such heavy responsibilities and are so closely concerned with the health of the people they serve, all states have strict laws about licensure. These may vary from state to state; the prospective pharmacist is instructed, while still in professional college, about the regulations applying in areas where he/she may wish to practice. All of the states require graduation from a program accredited by the Accreditation Council for Pharmacy Education (ACPE).

In order to receive a license, the pharmacist must pass an examination given by the Board of Pharmacy in the state where he/she plans to practice. Most states honor licenses issued by other states through a process of reciprocity coordinated by the National Association of Boards of Pharmacy.

Outlook for the Future

Community Pharmacy

Of the estimated 253,000 licensed pharmacists in the country, about 62% work in community pharmacies. Nearly everyone is familiar with community pharmacists and the pharmacy in which they practice.

You probably visit the community pharmacist more often than any other member of the health team. Americans make over five billion trips a year to pharmacies; the pharmacist has an opportunity to see at least one member of every family in his or her community every week. He or she talks to people when they are healthy and when they are sick, when they are "just browsing" or when they are concerned with an emergency, and when they are seeking advice or information. Pharmacists are playing an increasing role in the "wellness" movement, especially through counseling about preventive medicine and use of herbal products. According to one estimate, pharmacists get more than two billion inquiries a year from their patrons.

Advances in the use of technology in pharmacy practice now allow pharmacists to spend more time educating patients and maintaining and monitoring patient records. As a result, patients have come to depend on the pharmacist as a health care and information resource of the highest caliber.

Despite the variety of tasks performed in and out of the community pharmacy, pharmacists are specialists in the science and clinical use of medications. They must understand drug composition, chemical and physical properties, manufacture and uses, activity in the normal body as well as in the person who is ill, and must be familiar with tests for purity and for strength. Pharmacists are well-prepared to compound medicines and to dispense prescription orders written by physicians, dentists, and other prescribers. More and more prescribers rely on pharmacists for information about various medications, their availability and their activity, just as patrons do when they ask about nonprescription medicines.

If pharmacists want to combine their professional talents with the challenge of the fast-moving retail pharmacy business, they often consider management positions in chain pharmacy practice or ownership of their own pharmacy. In a community chain practice, career paths usually begin at the store level with subsequent advancement to positions at the district, regional, and corporate levels. Many chain companies have management development programs in marketing operations, legal affairs, third party programs, computerization, and pharmacy affairs. Pharmacists interested in supervisory or clinical experiences should consider a pharmacy residency or graduate study.

Independent retail practice offers the opportunity for pharmacists to be "their own boss." The spirit of entrepreneurship and motivation has enabled many pharmacists to successfully own their pharmacy or, through establishing consultation services, own their own pharmacy practice.

Hospitals and Other Institutional Settings

As society's health care needs have changed and expanded, there has been an increasing emphasis on provision of that care through organized health care settings. As a result, increasing numbers of pharmacists practice in large and small hospitals, nursing homes, extended care facilities, neighborhood health centers, and health maintenance organizations.

Hospital pharmacists, as members of the health care team along with physicians and nurses, have a unique opportunity for direct involvement with patient care. The clinical skills and knowledge of the contemporary pharmacist make this individual an authoritative source of drug information for physicians, nurses, and patients.

In addition to direct patient care involvement, pharmacists in hospitals are responsible for systems of total control of drug distribution, designed to assure that each patient receives the appropriate medication, in the correct form and dosage, at the correct time. Hospital pharmacists maintain records on each patient, using them not only to fill medication orders, but also to screen for drug allergies, drug interactions and adverse drug effects.

Contemporary hospital pharmacy practice includes a number of highly specialized areas, such as nuclear pharmacy, drug and poison information, and intravenous therapy. In addition, pharmacists provide specialized services in adult medicine, critical care, pediatrics, oncology, ambulatory care, and psychiatry. The nature and size of the hospital helps to determine the extent to which these specialized services are needed. Because of the diversity of activities involved in pharmacy departments, there is also an increasing demand for management expertise, including finance and budgeting, personnel administration, systems development, and planning.

About 23 percent of registered pharmacists work on a full- or part-time basis in hospitals or nursing homes. As hospital pharmacists continue to become more involved in providing patient-oriented services, the demand for practitioners in this area of pharmacy continues to grow.

Recent years have also seen dramatic growth in pharmacy services in managed health care, such as pharmacy benefit management companies and health maintenance organizations, and related organizations that offer coordinated ambulatory care by a multidisciplinary staff of health professionals, including pharmacists. In these settings, pharmacists provide primary leadership in the development of both clinical and administrative systems that manage and improve the use of medications.

Additional Opportunities in Pharmacy

Pharmacists are also employed by the U.S. Public Health Service, the Armed Forces, and the Department of Veteran Affairs (VA). Serving as commissioned officers, they can rise to the rank of colonel in the Army, and to equivalent ranks in the Public Health Service, the Navy, and the Air Force. In addition, pharmacists are employed by other governmental agencies, including the Food and Drug Administration (FDA), Centers for Disease Control and Prevention (CDC), National Institutes of Health (NIH), Indian Health Service (IHS), National Science Foundation (NSF), National Library of Medicine (NLM), and the U.S. Department of Health and Human Services.

The vast majority of the medicines pharmacists formerly compounded in their own pharmacies are now produced on a large scale by drug manufacturers. Pharmacists particularly interested in the scientific aspects of the profession can find challenging employment in the laboratories of academic institutions or pharmaceutical manufacturers. If research is a goal, pharmacy graduates usually go on to advanced study in pharmacy, pharmaceutics, pharmacology, toxicology, pharmaceutical chemistry, or other pharmaceutical sciences. A new field of research is pharmacy administration. Outcomes analysis, including cost-effectiveness of drug therapy, is one example of the kinds of issues fast becoming public policy concerns this discipline examines. All of these are examples of growing fields with excellent potential.

Future Prospects

Well-qualified pharmacists can be sure that the demand for their services will continue to increase in the future. They can also count on recognition for contributions to their community and to society.

Pharmacy has a direct relationship to pharmacology and other biophysical/biochemical sciences. Through the research activities of pharmaceutical manufacturers as well as of non-profit laboratories, the development of new medication therapies has become a major area of investigation and progress in the health-related sciences.

Career opportunities are available in community and hospital pharmacies, the military, in pharmaceutical research and manufacturing firms, nursing homes, public service agencies and in colleges and universities. Practice opportunities are excellent and promise to remain so.

Planning a Program of Study

General Information

All pharmacy colleges operate under one of three plans: (1) at least two years of college education followed by four academic years of professional study, (2) at least two years of college followed by three calendar years of professional study, or (3) an integrated curriculum for high school students who successfully complete the first 2-years of pre-professional study and are guaranteed admission into the professional pharmacy program. Where preprofessional education is required for admission, the two years of study must be taken in any accredited college or university. Due to the high number of applications, many pharmacy institutions give admissions preference to students who have previously earned a bachelor's degree.

In July 2000, the accreditation standard for the pharmacy degree became the Doctor of Pharmacy (Pharm.D.). Pharmacy schools no longer offer the B.S. in pharmacy degree. New students must graduate from an accredited Doctor of Pharmacy degree institution in order to be eligible to take the licensure examination of a state board of pharmacy and practice pharmacy in the U.S. Pharmacy colleges and schools are accredited by the Accreditation Council for Pharmacy Education (ACPE). A Pharm.D. degree requires at least four academic (or three calendar) years of professional study, following a minimum of two years of pre-pharmacy study, for a total of at least six years after high school. The majority of students enter a pharmacy program with 3 or more years of college experience. More than half of all student pharmacists have earned a bachelor's degree or higher prior to matriculation.

The Pharm.D. curriculum is designed to produce a scientifically and technically competent pharmacist who can apply this training in such a manner as to provide maximum health care services to patients. The Pharm.D. degree program provides students the opportunity to gain experience in patient-centered learning environments and to work in close cooperative relationships with health practitioners. The goal of pharmacy education is to prepare pharmacists who can assume expanded responsibilities in the care of patients and assure the provision of rational drug therapy and optimize health care outcomes.

Choice of Undergraduate Major

Undergraduate course work should include chemistry, biological and physical sciences, English or speech communications, social and behavioral sciences and the humanities. Courses in political science, accounting and finance are recommended as electives. Students are free to pick a major of their choosing or a specialized prepharmacy curriculum as long as all pharmacy course prerequisites are fulfilled. Prepharmacy requirements do vary by school and students are encouraged to carefully assess the requirements of the school(s) they wish to attend to ensure requisite course work is taken by the end of the fall term prior to enrollment. A summary of the course prerequisites required by each school is available on the AACP website (www.aacp.org) under the For Students and Applicants section.

The Admissions Process

Background

As of 2008, there were 110 colleges and schools of pharmacy in the United States and in Puerto Rico recognized by ACPE. The student should visit each pharmacy school website for information about admission requirements and deadlines. School-specific information is also available in the annual publication, *Pharmacy School Admission Requirements* (PSAR) offered online for free on the American Association of Colleges of Pharmacy (AACP) website at www.aacp.org.

In high school, students should select courses designed to prepare them for entrance to college. Courses in chemistry, biology, and physics are especially helpful in preparing students for the many college courses required for admission. Colleges of Pharmacy do not typically review high school transcripts in the professional pharmacy admissions process, but students are encouraged to do well in order to prepare for the rigor of the pharmacy curriculum.

PharmCAS

In 2008-2009 71 of all pharmacy degree programs in the U.S. participated in the Pharmacy College Application Service (PharmCAS) for admission. Through this centralized service applicants complete a single application and one set of official US and/or Canadian transcripts and references to apply to multiple Pharm.D. programs.

In addition to the PharmCAS application, pharmacy programs may require applicants to send a supplemental application and fee directly to the institution. The supplemental application deadline may be the same as the PharmCAS deadline, or at a later date. Students must complete all PharmCAS and school requirements before their application will be processed and reviewed.

PharmCAS is for first-year professional pharmacy degree applicants only. High school students, BS of Pharmacy degree graduates, and current student pharmacists who wish to transfer to another pharmacy degree program should contact institutions directly for application instructions. Visit the PharmCAS website at www.pharmcas.org to learn more about the admissions process and requirements.

Factors Evaluated by Admission Committees

Each pharmacy admissions office evaluates applications differently based on the institution's own criteria. Pharmacy schools may evaluate one or more of the following items for college students and graduates:

1. **Successful completion of pharmacy college course prerequisites**
   Students should complete most or all of the pharmacy course prerequisites by the end of the fall term prior to enrollment (e.g., Fall 2008 for 2009 entering class). Some pharmacy schools will consider applicants who complete prerequisites courses during the spring semester prior to enrollment.

2. **Cumulative undergraduate grade point average (GPA)**

   The minimum GPA requirement may be quite low as compared to the average GPA of applicants offered admission to a particular pharmacy school. Policies regarding forgiveness of repeated coursework vary by institution. For the 2008 entering class, the average overall undergraduate GPA was 3.46.

3. **Undergraduate science GPA**

   For the 2008 entering class, the average undergraduate science GPA was 3.33.

4. **Course prerequisite GPA**

   The minimum and average course prerequisite GPA varies significantly by institution.

5. **Class rank**

   Colleges and schools of pharmacy, in considering applicants for admission, may give attention to the relative position of students within their class-near the top, in the middle, or near the bottom. Colleges of pharmacy are interested in enrolling students who have demonstrated exceptional work in school and have the potential to contribute to the profession.

6. **PCAT test scores**

   Approximately three-fourths of all pharmacy colleges require or recommend that applicants take the Pharmacy College Admission Test (PCAT). For the 2008-09 examination cycle, this national exam will be administered four times a year and is designed to measure verbal and quantitative ability, reading comprehension, and biology and chemistry knowledge. Students should confer with the pharmacy colleges/schools to which they are interested in applying to ascertain the appropriate examination time, or visit with their health professions advisor who has experience and knowledge of pharmacy school admissions policies. For additional information on the PCAT, see your advisor or contact Pearson, Customer Relations-PCAT, 19500 Bulverde Road, San Antonio, TX 78259, (800) 622-3231, www.pcatweb.info.

7. **Letters of evaluation (recommendation)**

   Schools may require applicants to submit 1-4 letters of recommendation from particular individuals, such as a pharmacist, professor, or advisor. Selected pharmacy schools may require health professions advisors and evaluators to use a school-specific evaluation form in lieu of or in addition to the letter from the evaluator. PharmCAS collects electronic and paper letters letters of reference. School-specific information about evaluator types accepted is available on the PharmCAS website. Go to www.pharmcas.org/docs/ReqTypebySchool.pdf.

8. **Results of applicant interviews**

   All pharmacy schools will require competitive applicants to visit the campus for an in-person interview. Applicants who have researched and gained direct exposure to the profession will be better prepared to respond to the interview questions. Applicants may be rated on communication skills, professional behavior, knowledge of the profession, critical thinking skills, and motivation to pursue a career in pharmacy.

9. **Written communication skills via an essay exercise during interview process**

   Pharmacy schools may assess an applicant's writing skills through an on-campus essay exercise or by examining the applicant's PCAT score on the writing subtest.

10. **Volunteer or paid experience working with patients in a pharmacy or health-related setting (hospital, nursing home, etc.)**

Pharmacy colleges encourage or require applicants to have volunteer or paid experience working with patients in a pharmacy or health-related setting. On-going work or volunteer experience in a pharmacy setting may be an important factor in the admissions process. If students are unable to gain work or volunteer experience directly related to pharmacy due to state law restrictions or availability, they should contact their selected pharmacy admission offices to determine what other experiences are accepted.

11. **Professionalism attributes demonstrated by portfolio or extracurricular experiences**

Pharmacy schools may require applicants to document activities that demonstrate their professional dispositions and potential.

12. **Residency status (if a state-supported public institution)**

Some U.S. pharmacy institutions give preference to in-state (resident) students. Out-of-state (non-resident) and foreign applicants may vie for a limited number of positions or may be ineligible for admission, depending on institutional and state policies. Private pharmacy institutions may offer out-of-state and foreign applicants a greater number of positions within the program as compared to state-supported, public institutions.

13. **Diversity of background (as defined by the institution)**

Resources

1. *Pharmacy School Admissions Requirements*, American Association of Colleges of Pharmacy, 1727 King Street, Alexandria, VA 22314-2841; 703/739-2330; www.aacp.org; www.pharmcas.org; www.ajpe.org For a complete listing of the 110 pharmacy schools, visit this website: www.aacp.org.

2. Career Information Specific to a Particular Practice Setting: American Pharmacists Association, 1100 15th Street NW, Suite 400, Washington, DC 20037, www.pharmacist.com/students.

3. American Association of Pharmaceutical Scientists, 2107 Wilson Blvd, Suite 700, Arlington, VA 22201-3042. www.aaps.org.

4. American Society of Health System Pharmacists, 7272 Wisconsin Avenue, Bethesda, MD 20814, www.ashp.org.

   National Association of Chain Drug Stores, P.O. Box 1417-D49, 413 North Lee Street, Alexandria, VA 22313, www.nacds.org.

   National Community Pharmacists Association (represents independent retail pharmacists), 205 Daingerfield Road, Alexandria, VA 22314, www.ncpanet.org.

   American Society of Consultant Pharmacists, 1321 Duke Street, Alexandria, VA 22314, www.ascp.com.

   National Association of Boards of Pharmacy (Licensing Information), 700 Busse Highway, Park Ridge, IL 60068, www.nabp.net.

   Program Accreditation Information: Accreditation Council for Pharmacy Education, 20 North Clark Street, Suite 2500 Chicago, IL 60602-5109, info@acpe-accredit.org, www.acpe-accredit.org.

PHYSICAL THERAPY (P.T.)

General Description

Physical therapists (PTs) are experts in movement and function of the body. Physical therapists provide services that help restore function, improve mobility, relieve pain, and prevent or limit permanent physical disabilities associated with injury or disease. Patient examinations in physical therapy include, but are not limited to, testing of muscle function, strength, joint flexibility, range of motion, balance and coordination, posture, respiration, skin integrity, motor function, quality of life, and activities of daily living. Physical therapists also determine a patient's ability to reintegrate into the workforce or community after illness or injury. Once an examination is complete and a diagnosis has been determined, the physical therapist designs a plan of care that includes short and long-term functional goals and interventions that may include, but not be limited to, exercise, traction, mobilization/manual therapy, ultrasound and/or electrotherapy, vestibular training, motor learning and development, and patient and family education. Interventions will often include the use of assistive and adaptive devices such as crutches, wheelchairs, orthotics, and prosthetics. An important component of physical therapist patient management involves teaching the patient appropriate ways to move or perform particular tasks to prevent further injury and to promote health and wellness.

Physical therapists practice in a variety of settings including hospitals, clinics, private physical therapy offices, home health agencies, skilled nursing facilities, rehabilitation centers, school systems, sports medicine facilities, industrial settings, academic settings (education and research), and government agencies. About two-thirds of physical therapists are employed in private outpatient offices or group practices, health system or hospital-based outpatient facility, hospitals, or academic institutions. Designated areas with board specialty certification for physical therapists include cardiovascular and pulmonary, clinical electrophysiology, geriatrics, neurology, orthopaedics, pediatrics, sports physical therapy, and women's health. Additional areas of focused clinical practice for physical therapists include acute care, aquatic physical therapy, education and clinical education, hand rehabilitation, health policy and administration, home health, oncology, research, private practice, and veteran's affairs.

Physical Therapist Practice

All states require physical therapists to have graduated from an accredited physical therapist educational program as well as pass a national licensure examination. Physical therapist practice is governed by state licensure laws and as such there may be additional requirements and fees beyond the required national licensure examination to practice in a specific state or jurisdiction.

Outlook for the Future

Vision 2020

Physical therapy is a dynamic and progressive profession that is intentionally shaped by a focused vision. In 2000, the governing body for the profession approved Vision 2020 in physical therapy. This Vision serves to provide short, intermediate, and long-term guidance and direction for the profession. The Vision statement states that:

> "Physical therapy, by 2020, will be provided by physical therapists who are doctors of physical therapy and who may be board-certified specialists. Consumers will have direct access to physical therapists in all environments for patient/client management, prevention, and wellness services. Physical therapists will be practitioners of choice in patients'/clients' health networks and will hold all privileges of autonomous practice. Physical therapists may be assisted by physical therapist assistants who are educated and licensed to provide physical therapist directed and supervised components of interventions.

Guided by integrity, life-long learning, and a commitment to comprehensive and accessible health programs for all people, physical therapists and physical therapist assistants will render evidence-based services throughout the continuum of care and improve quality of life for society. They will provide culturally sensitive care distinguished by trust, respect, and an appreciation for individual differences. While fully availing themselves of new technologies, as well as basic and clinical research, physical therapists will continue to provide direct patient/client care. They will maintain active responsibility for the growth of the physical therapy profession and the health of the people it serves."

The six elements that are described in the Vision 2020 Statement include the Doctor of Physical Therapy, Evidenced-based Practice, Autonomous Practice, Direct Access, Practitioner of Choice, and Professionalism. These six elements are critical to the future direction of the practice of physical therapy as well as how practitioners will be providing evidenced-based and patient-centered care. Thus, potential applicants should thoughtfully consider the role and responsibilities of the physical therapist within the framework of Vision 2020, given that this vision will guide the future direction of the profession and the individual practitioner within the profession.

Employment Projections

Although federal legislation limiting therapy reimbursement has increased competition for jobs in the past few years, the U.S. Department of Labor, Bureau of Labor Statistics (BLS) projects that the employment of physical therapists is expected to grow faster than the average. In fact, the BLS lists physical therapy as one of the 30 fastest growing occupations through 2012 with a projected growth of 35%. In 2006, the median annual earnings of physical therapists by geographic region were between $70,000 and $80,000 and the median gross annual earned income of PTs by highest earned degree fluctuated between $60,000 (Professional DPT) and $85,000 (PhD or equivalent). Variation in income is dependent upon years of practice experience, geographical location, employment setting, highest earned academic degree, and supervisory responsibility.

Professional Development Opportunities

A myriad of opportunities are available to licensed physical therapists for continued and ongoing lifelong professional development. These opportunities include, but are not limited to, pursuing clinical mastery in practice by completing an approved clinical residency or clinical fellowship, pursuit of clinical specialization in 8 specialty areas through the American Board of Physical Therapy Specialties, furthering one's formal academic education (e.g., PhD, DScPT, ScD, DPTSc) in preparation for conducting research and teaching in an academic setting, advancing within clinical practice through additional programs that offer practice credentials, and completing continuing education courses provided through web-based distance learning, home study, and conferences offered nationally, regionally, and locally.

Planning a Program of Study

Physical Therapist Education Preparation

All professional (entry-level) physical therapist educational programs currently award a postbaccalaureate degree, which includes either a master's or clinical doctoral (DPT) degree upon completion of the program. In 2008, there were 214 accredited and developing PT programs in the U.S. (210 accredited; 4 developing). As of December 10, 2008 of the 210 accredited programs, 196 (93.3%) awarded the DPT degree and 14 (6.7%) awarded the masters degree. Physical therapist professional programs have reported (99.5%) their intent to award the DPT degree by 2013. Specific physical therapist educational programs on the APTA web directory can be accessed at www.apta.org, and then click on PT programs.

The vast majority of PT educational programs require applicants to possess a bachelor's degree along with the successful completion of specific prerequisites that can vary from one academic program to another. The undergraduate degree earned varies as long as the prerequisite coursework is completed along with the major course of study. Some of the undergraduate degrees earned in preparation for admission to a physical therapist program include, but are not limited to, biology, chemistry, physics, exercise physiology, exercise science, psychology, anthropology, and others.

Although requirements for physical therapist programs currently vary by academic institution, prerequisite requirements common to a majority of programs typically may include (but are not limited to): biology, anatomy, physiology, chemistry, physics, statistics, psychology, and other social sciences. Many PT programs also require some paid or unpaid experience in at least one, if not more, physical therapy settings. Applicants also are required to take the Graduate Record Exam (GRE). Information on this computerized exam can be found at www.gre.org.

Entry into physical therapist programs is competitive. As of March 2007, approval was provided to begin the development of a Centralized Application Service for application to professional (entry-level) physical therapist programs.

Students seeking entry into a PT program should have a clear picture of the profession and the broad spectrum of opportunities that are available. As indicated previously, volunteer or paid experiences are often required by programs for admission. The purpose of these physical therapy exposures is for the applicant to have an opportunity to personally explore the profession with its rewards and challenges, interact with physical therapists regarding their impressions about their roles and responsibilities within health care, and to determine if physical therapy is a good "fit" for the applicant. In addition, APTA's website offers information for prospective students including Frequently Asked Questions, Directory of Accredited PT Programs, Scholarship/Financial Aid, Your Career in Physical Therapy, and PT Demographics. To access this information, refer to www.apta.org/Students/Information for Prospective PT and PTA students.

Personal Attributes

Students seeking entry into a physical therapist program should possess attributes that include, but are not limited to, strong interpersonal, communication, problem solving, critical thinking, and leadership skills, along with a sincere desire to enter a helping health care profession. Students should also be interested in providing physical therapy services to patients of all ages throughout the continuum of care. Provision of these services may range from patients with acutely ill conditions, through rehabilitation, and management of chronic conditions. Likewise, students should also be interested in improving the health and wellness of patients while preventing future injury or disability. In addition, applicants should be able to demonstrate behavior reflective of and integral to the profession's core values that include accountability, altruism, caring/compassion, excellence, integrity, professional duty, and social responsibility.

Program Application

There is a new application service, the Physical Therapist Centralized Application Service (PTCAS), available for students applying to CAPTE accredited physical therapist programs as of August 1, 2008. Currently 72 physical therapist programs use this service for their applicants and is anticipated that the number of programs will continue to increase in the coming year. To access a list of academic programs that use this service, refer to the PTCAS Directory at www.ptcas.org/Directory.html. PTCAS allows physical therapist applicants to use a single Web-based application and one set of materials to apply to multiple physical therapist professional programs. PTCAS is a service of the American Physical Therapy Association (APTA) and is administered by Liaison International (LI), an education information technology company located in Watertown, Massachusetts. PTCAS will offer a secure online Advisor Portal in 2009 to NAAHP members and other advisors authorized by participating programs that will allow users to track the status and success rates of their students.

Resources

American Physical Therapy Association (APTA)
1111 North Fairfax Street
Alexandria, VA 22314-1488
703/684-2782 or 800/999-2782
www.apta.org

PT Accredited Program Information
For a complete list of the 210 accredited physical therapist programs, visit www.apta.org/AM/
Template.cfm?Section=CAPTE3&Template=/aptaapps/accreditedschools/
acc_schools_map.cfm&process=3&type=PT.

2007-2008 Fact Sheet, Physical Therapist Education Programs, Department of Accreditation, American Physical
Therapy Association. Alexandria, Va: May 2008. www.apta.org/AM/
Template.cfm?Section=PT_Programs3&CONTENTID=43471&TEMPLATE=/CM/ContentDisplay.cfm

Number of PT and PTA Programs. Department of Accreditation. American Physical Therapy Association.
Alexandria, Va: December 2008.
www.apta.org/AM/Template.cfm?Section=PT_Programs3&CONTENTID=45221&TEMPLATE=/CM/
ContentDisplay.cfm

PTCAS
For more information about and a listing or programs that use the PTCAS, visit www.ptcas.org

Demographics and Statistics
2007 PT Member Demographic Profile. American Physical Therapy Association. Alexandria, Va: June 2007.
www.apta.org/AM/Template.cfm?Section=Demographics&Template=/TaggedPage/
TaggedPageDisplay.cfm&TPLID=101&ContentID=14332

U.S. Department of Labor
Bureau of Labor Statistics
Occupational Outlook Handbook 2004-2005
www.bls.gov/oco

PHYSICIAN ASSISTANT (P.A.)

General Description

Physician assistants (PAs) are licensed health professionals who practice medicine with physician supervision as members of a medical team. PAs deliver a broad range of medical and surgical services to diverse populations in rural and urban settings. As part of their comprehensive responsibilities, PAs conduct physical exams, diagnose and treat illnesses, order and interpret tests, counsel on preventive health care, assist in surgery, and prescribe medications. A PA's scope of practice varies, based on training, experience, and state law. A PA's clinical responsibilities correspond to the supervising physician's practice, so in general, a physician assistant will see many of the same types of patients as the physician.

The PA profession is relatively new compared to other health professions, having been founded in the mid-1960s. At the beginning of 2008, there were more than 68,000 physician assistants in clinical practice. PA educational programs graduated approximately 4,600 new graduates in 2007. While PAs continue their traditional role of bringing health care to the underserved in rural and inner city areas, today they practice in all urban, suburban, and rural settings. According to the 2008 census survey conducted by the American Academy of Physician Assistants (AAPA), 15 percent of clinically practicing PAs work primarily in non-metropolitan areas. According to the 2008 census survey, 37 percent of respondents reported that their medical specialty was one of the primary care fields: family/general practice medicine (26%), general internal medicine (5%), obstetrics/gynecology (2%), and general pediatrics (3%). Twenty-five percent of respondents reported they work in general surgery or a surgical subspecialty.

Outlook for the Future

The PA profession will grow much faster than the average occupation in the decade 2006 through 2016, according to the Bureau of Labor Statistics' (BLS) most recent employment projections. The BLS predicts that total employment for PAs is projected to increase by 27 percent during these years. The PA profession has consistently been listed as one of the fastest-growing occupations by the BLS. For more information on BLS economic and employment projections, go to www.bls.gov.

Planning a Program

For many years the number of PA educational programs remained fairly constant, but beginning in the mid-1990s their numbers have increased dramatically. There are now 142 programs that have been awarded accreditation by the Accreditation Review Commission on Education for the Physician Assistant (ARC-PA). The ARC-PA is the only accrediting body for PA programs. To be accredited, programs must meet its stringent academic and professional requirements.

Although PA programs vary in their missions, requirements, and admissions processes, almost all require applicants to have previous health care experience. Many applicants bring health care experience from previous careers as an emergency medical technician, orderly or a nurse's aide, nurse, x-ray technician, respiratory therapist, or military corpsman. This experience might also include volunteering a substantial number of hours in a hospital or clinic.

Most programs are looking for people with life experience as well as medical experience, and most require that applicants have a minimum of two years of college credits in addition to the health care-related experience described above.

Coursework to be completed before applying to PA programs differs according to the entrance requirements for each program, but generally includes biology, English, humanities, social sciences, chemistry, college math, and psychology. Courses in anatomy, pharmacology, biochemistry, physical and clinical diagnosis, physiology, microbiology, and clinical medicine are typical during the first year of PA programs, which is usually classroom-based. Second-year students rotate through the various specialties, which include obstetrics/gynecology, surgery, orthopedics, and geriatrics, in addition to other specialties with a primary care focus.

Following graduation from an accredited program, graduates are required to pass a national certifying examination developed by the independent National Commission on Certification of Physician Assistants in cooperation with the National Board of Medical Examiners. To maintain certification, individuals must log 100 hours of continuing medical education every two years and pass a recertification exam every six years. In addition to passing the exam, PAs are licensed by the state in which they practice.

Admissions Process

Acceptance to a PA program is competitive. The Central Application Service for Physician Assistants (CASPA) represents approximately 76 percent of all PA programs. According to CASPA, there were 2.75 applicants for each PA program seat for the class entering in 2008. Figures from the Physician Assistant Education Association's *Annual Report on Physician Assistant Education Programs in the United States, 2007-2008 (not published as of winter 2009)*, showed that the proportion of students with bachelor's degrees stays at 76 percent this year, and up more than 15 points since 2000. The average number of entering class students in these accredited programs is between 43-44, and the average length of training is 26-27 months.

According to the annual report on PA programs for 2007-2008, the proportion of enrollees who are female is 72 percent. Over the past decade, this percentage increased steadily and has remained stable for the past three years. PA classes have long been predominately female.

Competitive applicants for PA programs have completed the prerequisite coursework required by the specific schools to which they are applying. They also present a solid understanding of the profession and patient care, demonstrated by significant health-related experience. Many of the PA programs require applicants to take the Graduate Record Exam (GRE). Letters of recommendation from teachers, employers, and others are also part of the admissions process.

PAs are considered essential partners in America's medical workforce. As the country faces a growing demand for health care services, the mix of physicians, physician assistants, and other providers will be redefined to meet the structure of emerging practices.

Resources

Physician Assistant Education Association
300 N. Washington Street
Alexandria, VA 22314
(703) 548-5538
www.PAEAonline.org

American Academy of Physician Assistants
950 N. Washington Street
Alexandria, VA 22314
(703) 836-2272
www.aapa.org

U.S. Department of Labor
Bureau of Labor Statistics
www.bls.gov/oco

PODIATRIC MEDICINE (D.P.M.)

General Description

Podiatric medicine is a branch of the medical sciences devoted to the study of human movement, with the medical care of the foot and ankle as its primary focus. A doctor of podiatric medicine is to the foot what a dentist is to the mouth or an optometrist to the eye — a specialist who has undergone lengthy, thorough study to become uniquely well-qualified to treat a specific part of the body.

A Doctor of Podiatric Medicine (DPM) specializes in the prevention, diagnosis, and treatment of foot disorders, diseases and injuries. Podiatric Physicians makes independent judgments and performs or orders all necessary diagnostic tests. They perform surgery; administer medications, including DEA-restricted medications; and prescribe physical therapy regimens.

The Doctor of Podiatric Medicine often detects serious health problems that may otherwise go unnoticed because of symptoms first expressed in problems of the lower extremity such as diabetes, arthritis, heart disease, or kidney disease. These doctors are educated in state-of-the-art techniques involving surgery, orthopedics, dermatology, physical medicine and rehabilitation.

Podiatrists work in general or group practices and are free to develop a practice specialty such as pediatrics, geriatrics, or sports medicine. In addition to private practice, they serve on the staffs of hospitals and long-term care facilities, on the faculties of schools of medicine and nursing, in the armed forces as commissioned officers, in the U.S. Public Health Service, and in municipal health departments.

The degree of Doctor of Podiatric Medicine (D.P.M.) is awarded after four years of study at one of eight accredited podiatric medical colleges. The colleges differ in size and location, although the curriculum leading to the D.P.M. degree is quite similar at each institution. The first two years concentrate on classroom instruction and laboratory work in the basic medical sciences. Medical education for all physicians is characterized by course work in the basic sciences, including anatomy, physiology, biochemistry, pharmacology, microbiology, pathology, immunology, etc. In addition, the student of podiatric medicine also learns the fundamentals of specialized medicine, which include biomechanics, lower extremity anatomy, podiatric pathology, infectious diseases, orthopedics, and sports medicine courses. The third and fourth years of study focus on the clinical sciences and patient care. However clinical exposure begins as early as the first year. Experience is gained in some of the finest clinics in the country, which include community clinics, hospitals, and professional office settings.

After completing four years of podiatric medical education, graduates select a Podiatric Medicine and Surgery Residency of twenty-four or thirty-six months in duration. Although the podiatric physician is required by nearly all states to complete a minimum of one year of postgraduate residency training in an approved healthcare institution, two years are required for board certification. A podiatric residency provides an interdisciplinary experience with rotations such as anesthesiology, internal medicine, infectious disease, surgery, orthopedics, pediatrics and emergency medicine. The thirty-six month residency includes extensive training in rear foot and ankle surgery. The AACPM assists students in the national, centralized application and residency matching process known as CASPR, in which all entry-level residency programs are required to participate. This service, modeled after the NRMP, helps students to save time and money during their residency search.

Podiatric physicians are licensed in all 50 states, the District of Columbia and Puerto Rico to treat the foot and its related or governing structures by medical, surgical or other means. State licensing requirements generally include graduation from one of the eight accredited colleges of podiatric medicine, passage of the National Board exams, which are taken in two parts while in podiatric medical school, and postgraduate training, as well as written and oral examinations. Podiatric physicians may also become certified in one or both specialty areas: primary medicine and orthopedics, or surgery.

The Decision to Pursue Podiatric Medicine

Students who do well in the basic sciences and are interested in becoming integral members of the health care team should seriously consider a career in podiatric medicine. Podiatrists are often able to provide immediate patient relief and are able to detect serious health problems early because of their specialized training. Preventing serious illness or identifying potential problems while still in treatable stages can be most satisfying. The independence afforded any practicing physician who chooses to be self-employed is another attractive feature of this profession.

In general, the practice of podiatric medicine lends itself to flexible hours and is therefore comfortable for individuals who want time for family, friends and other involvements that characterize a balanced lifestyle. The work hours of a podiatric physician can vary from 30 to 60 hours a week.

Earnings of podiatrists depend upon geographic location, type of practice, number of patients seen per week, years of experience, etc. According to a survey by the American Podiatric Medical Association (APMA 2006 Podiatric Practice Survey), the average <u>NET</u> income of full-time (30+ hrs. /week) podiatric physicians in 2006 was as follows:

Net income range (after practice expenses) in 2006	Percentage of podiatrists with that level of income in 2006
Less than $25,000	2%
$25,000 - $75,000	11%
$76,000 - $100,000	13%
$101,000 - $150,000	25%
$151,000 - $200,000	17%
$201,000 - $250,000	12%
$251,000 – 300,000	8%
More than $300,000	13%

The average net income increased from an estimated $108,000 in 1995 and $111,000 in 1997 to $134,000 in 2001, $154,000 in 2004 and $189,030 in 2006.

Planning a Program of Study

Like other fields of medicine, the schools and colleges of podiatric medicine accept students from any major provided that they have completed course work that fulfills the science prerequisites. Many students enter podiatric medicine from other health professions, such as nursing, pharmacy, clinical laboratory science (formerly medical technology) and physical therapy. Candidates for admission should present evidence of strong preparation for professional study. The minimum requirement for admission is completion of three academic years (90 semester hours) of study at an accredited college or university. The vast majority of students who matriculate, however, have completed a bachelor's degree.

The minimum course requirements for admission to the colleges of podiatric medicine are as follows:

Biology	8 semester hours or 12 quarter hours
General Inorganic Chemistry	8 semester hours or 12 quarter hours
Organic Chemistry	8 semester hours or 12 quarter hours
Physics	8 semester hours or 12 quarter hours
English	6 semester hours or 9 quarter hours

All science courses must include laboratory work. These courses should be completed by the end of the junior year, as they are good preparation for the standardized admissions tests, which should be taken before starting the senior year of college, if the applicant plans to enroll in podiatric school right after college. Students may complete a request form at the AACPM website: www.aacpm.org to receive a "College Information Booklet" that lists each college's admission requirements, or utilize the direct links at the website to the colleges of podiatric medicine.

Interested applicants should visit the office of a practicing podiatrist to learn more about the profession and possibly to obtain a letter of recommendation. An applicant can access the DPM Mentors Network at the AACPM website to contact a podiatrist in his/her state for shadowing purposes or information about the practice of podiatric medicine. Visiting a podiatric practice both demonstrates an applicant's seriousness in applying to a college of podiatric medicine and gives an opportunity for the student to see first-hand if the profession fits his or her needs and aptitudes. A letter of recommendation or a statement made by the podiatrist can document evidence of this experience. To find a mentor, go to www.aacpm.org and click on the "Find a Mentor" tab. Select a state and a list of both podiatric physicians and current students will appear for your use.

The Admissions Process

The Application Service

The American Association of Colleges of Podiatric Medicine administers the application service, E-AACPMAS, which processes all applications submitted for admission to its member colleges of podiatric medicine. E-AACPMAS enables applicants to apply simultaneously to any number of the eight member colleges by submitting just one application. To complete the web application, interested students should go directly to www.e-aacpmas.org. A correctly completed web application will be processed and digitally transmitted to the applicant's designated college(s) within 24 hours after receipt by AACPMAS.

Standardized Admissions Tests

All students are required to submit scores from a graduate-level standardized admissions test prior to matriculation, such as, MCAT, DAT, GRE, etc. Candidates should consult with each school to determine which test(s) is (are) acceptable for admission consideration. The following chart provides a breakdown of the acceptable standardized tests:

COLLEGES OF PODIATRIC MEDICINE
Acceptable Standardized Tests

SCHOOL	Standardized Tests Accepted During the 2009 AACPMAS Cycle
AZPod	MCAT Last MCAT test date: 5/28/09
BUSPM	MCAT, DAT Last MCAT test date: 6/18/09
CSPM	MCAT Last MCAT test date: 7/2/09
CPMS	MCAT Last MCAT test date: 6/18/09
NYCPM	MCAT, DAT Last MCAT test date: 6/18/09
OCPM	MCAT Last MCAT test date: 7/2/09
SCPM	MCAT Last MCAT test date: 5/2809
TUSPM	MCAT, DAT, GRE Last MCAT test date: 7/17/09

Results of these standardized admission tests taken more than three years prior to year of application are *NOT* acceptable. For fall admission, applicants are advised to take the MCAT no later than spring of the year of application. Scores on the MCAT must be sent to the American Association of Colleges of Podiatric Medicine Application Service (AACPMAS). Test results for the GRE and DAT must be sent *directly* to the colleges.

Official Transcripts

Official transcripts from each undergraduate school attended must be sent _directly_ to all of the colleges of podiatric medicine to which the applicant applies. Transcripts are not to be sent to AACPMAS.

The Letters of Evaluation

Each of the colleges of podiatric medicine has different requirements for letters of recommendation. Typically, letters are requested from a pre-professional advisory committee or from members of the science faculty at a college or university. At least one recommendation from a podiatrist is usually requested. Letters of recommendation are to be mailed _directly_ to the individual colleges of podiatric medicine. Applicants need to contact each college for their specific requirements for letters of recommendation. Each college is directly linked from the AACPM's website at www.aacpm.org.

The Interview

Each institution invites qualified applicants for a personal interview conducted by the Admissions Committee at that school. The interview is considered to be an important tool for making final admissions decisions. For more information on interviewing, refer to chapter 2.

Resources

1. _"Podiatric Medicine as a Career — What is a DPM?"_ brochure published by the American Association of Colleges of Podiatric Medicine, www.aacpm.org 15850 Crabbs Branch Way, Suite 320, Rockville, MD 20855; 800-922-9266; inside Maryland: 301-948-0957, X-21.

2. _AACPMAS College Information Booklet._ Published by AACPM (see address above).

3. Catalogs and other resource materials from AACPM's member colleges which are linked from AACPM's website at: www.aacpm.org.

4. _"Podiatric Medicine: A Career that Fits Your Future"_ brochure published by the American Podiatric Medical Association (APMA), www.apma.org 9312 Old Georgetown Road, Bethesda, MD 20814-1698; 301-571-9200.

   Inquiries about podiatric medicine can be directed to the association by email: aacpmas@aacpm.org by writing: AACPM, 15850 Crabbs Branch Way, Suite 320, Rockville, MD 20855; or by calling: 800-922-9266 or inside Maryland: 301-948-0957, X-21. For a complete list of the eight colleges of podiatric medicine, visit www.aacpm.org.

PUBLIC HEALTH (M.P.H.)

General Description

In the fall of 2001, the nation was confronted by several tragic events that underscored its lack of preparation for the unthinkable. In the aftermath of these events, public health professionals emerged to do precisely what they were trained to do — provide crisis leadership, investigate immediate risks to the public's health, prevent further risk exposure, and reassure a concerned public.

Lately, it seems that public health issues face us every day and in every area of the world. Front-page headlines present society with public health issues on a daily basis: emerging infectious diseases such as SARS, making its way from China to Canada and the United States; prescription drug benefits under Medicare; the increase of HIV-AIDS among young heterosexual women and its spread in South Africa; the increase of childhood obesity and the concomitant increase in type II diabetes among children; the impact of adolescent pregnancy; and, the ongoing social, economic and health disasters related Hurricane Katrina. These are all public health challenges.

Three things can be said about public health: it is relevant, it is challenging, and it is necessary. The mission of public health is the "fulfillment of society's interest in assuring the conditions in which people can be healthy" (Institute of Medicine, The Future of Public Health). The most important aspect of public health is that it focuses on the health and well being of populations. While medicine is concerned with individual patients, public health regards the community as its patient.

What are the functions of public health? According to the Public Health Functions Project site (www.health.gov/phfunctions/public.htm), public health:
- Prevents epidemics and the spread of disease
- Protects against environmental hazards
- Prevents injuries
- Promotes and encourages healthy behaviors
- Responds to disasters and assists communities in recovery
- Assures the quality and accessibility of health services

In fact, during the twentieth century, the average lifespan of individuals in the United States lengthened by thirty years. Twenty- five of this gain is attributable to advances in public health such as assuring clean water, immunizing children against infectious diseases, improving motor vehicle safety, creating safer workplaces, controlling infectious diseases, providing safer and healthier foods, providing prenatal care and well child care to ensure healthier mothers and babies, and developing major campaigns to stop smoking.

Public health professionals can be basic scientists researching new viruses, health educators who work with teenage moms or who develop anti-smoking campaigns, or epidemiologists who study the emergence, frequency and geographic spread of West Nile Virus or the risk factors associated with certain cancers. They can also be biostatisticians who run clinical trials for pharmaceutical companies or work with a team to determine the impact of genetics on certain diseases, or hospital administrators or health policy experts who write or evaluate federal health legislation. Additionally, they can be health researchers who study outcomes of cardiac surgery or determinants of access to health care, or sanitarians or environmental researchers who determine the impact of car emissions on the public's health. Public health professionals come from a wide range of disciplines, work in a variety of settings and have many professions such as nursing, dentistry, medicine, law, social work, environmental sciences or may have a sole degree in public health.

More information about the field of public health can be found at: www.whatispublichealth.org, a website designed to guide interested students and advisors alike about the public health profession. This website includes an interactive game "Outbreak at Water's Edge," vignettes from public health professionals, an online quiz can be taken multiple times, video files and examples of public health in action.

Outlook for the Future

The demand today for public health professionals is great and is increasing in the face of new threats, new knowledge, and new demands. The opportunities are as wide and varied as the public health challenges facing society.

Public health takes place in many different career settings. The following are examples of professional career tracks in public health. Public health professionals find career tracks in many professional settings such as a researcher in a laboratory, an administrative official in a public or private organization, a teacher in an educational institution, or a policy analyst with a national think-tank.

Environmental Health

Environmental health deals with the air we breathe, the water we drink, the complex interactions between human genetics and our surroundings. These environmental risk factors can cause diseases such as asthma, cancer, and food poisoning. Environmental health studies the impact of our surroundings on our health.

Biostatistics

Biostatistics uses data analysis to determine the cause of disease and injuries, as well as to identify health trends within communities. This field entails collecting and studying information, forecasting scenarios, and making reliable conclusions. Biostatistics involves estimating the number of deaths from gun violence or looking at trends in drunk driving injuries by using math and science.

Behavioral Sciences/Health Education

Behavioral science/health education is concerned with stopping the spread of sexually transmitted diseases, such as herpes and HIV/AIDS; helping youth recognize the dangers of binge drinking; and promoting seatbelt use. Behavioral Science/Health Education focuses on ways that encourage people to make healthy choices. This includes the development of community-wide education programs that range from promoting healthy lifestyles to preventing disease and injury, to researching complex health issues.

Epidemiology

Epidemiology is used when food poisoning or an influenza outbreak attacks a community. In that situation, "disease detectives" or epidemiologists are asked to investigate the cause of disease and control its spread. Epidemiologists do fieldwork to determine what causes disease or injury, what the risks are, who is at risk, and how to prevent further incidences. They understand the demographic and social trends upon disease and injury. The initial discovery and containment of an outbreak, such as West Nile virus, often come from epidemiologists, as well as the initial determination of the relationship between smoking and lung cancer.

Health Services Administration

Health services administration entails managing the database at a school clinic, developing budgets for a health department, creating policies for health insurance companies, and directing hospital services. The field of health services administration combines politics, business, and science in managing the human and fiscal resources needed to deliver effective public health services.

Maternal and Child Health

Maternal and child health involves providing information and access to birth control, promoting the health of a pregnant woman and an unborn child, and dispensing vaccinations to children. Professionals in maternal and child health improve the public health delivery systems specifically for women, children, and their families through advocacy, education, and research.

Nutrition

Nutrition requires promoting healthy eating and regular exercise, researching the effect of diet on the elderly, and teaching the dangers of overeating and overdieting. This field examines how food and nutrients affect the wellness and lifestyle of population. Nutrition encompasses the combination of education and science to promote health and disease prevention.

International/Global Health

International/global health addresses health concerns from a global perspective and encompasses all areas of public health (e.g., biostatistics, epidemiology, nutrition, maternal and child health, etc.). International health professionals address health concerns among different cultures in countries worldwide.

Public Health Laboratory Practice

Public health laboratory professionals perform tests on biological and environmental samples in order to diagnose, prevent, treat, and control infectious diseases in communities; to ensure the safety of our food and water; to screen for the presence of certain diseases within communities; and to respond to public health emergencies, such as bioterrorism.

Public Health Degree Programs

The most common public health degree is the Master of Public Health (MPH); however, most schools offer other master's degrees, such as the Master of Health Administration (MHA) or Master of Science (M.S.) Additionally, all accredited schools of public health must offer a doctoral degree, such as the Ph.D., Doctorate of Public Health (DrPH) or Doctorate of Science (D.Sc.).

Professional degrees generally have a greater orientation towards practice in public health settings. The MPH, DrPH, and MHA are examples of degrees that are geared towards those who want careers as practitioners of public health in traditional health departments, managed care organizations, community-based organizations, hospitals, consulting firms, international agencies, and state and federal agencies, among others.

Academic degrees are more oriented toward students wishing to seek a career in academics and research rather than public health practice. Examples of academic degrees are the M.S., Ph.D., and Sc.D.. However, each school of public health can tailor its degree programs significantly, so students are encouraged to check with individual schools for more information.

In an effort to ensure a well-rounded education, all MPH students are required to take at least one course in the five core areas of public health: biostatistics, epidemiology, environmental health, behavioral sciences/health education, and health services administration. Students take the rest of their courses either in their area of specialization or they may take additional credits in other areas such as maternal and child health, nutrition, genomics, informatics, and public health law. There is a rich menu of choices for a student to choose from when enrolling in a school of public health. First year students are encouraged to take the five core courses early on because many students find unexpected interest in another concentration. Most master's programs are generally two years in length for full-time students, though executive programs for students with significant public health experience can be completed in less time. Doctoral programs are normally three to five years in length.

Public health is an interdisciplinary field — not only does it require specialists in public health, but it also requires the cooperation and participation of other professionals, such as medical doctors, lawyers, dentists, nurses, urban planners, etc. To this end, there are over 45 joint degrees in public health, which include the MD/MPH, JD/MPH, MPH/MBA and the MPH/MSW. Joint degrees are an excellent opportunity for students who want to practice the clinical health professions while applying public health principles.

The salary ranges, as follows, are the actual salaries earned (adjusted for inflation using the national CPI — Bureau of Labor Statistics) within one year of graduation as reported by the most recent nationwide survey of graduates conducted by ASPH:

Biostatistics	$33,000 – $63,000
Epidemiology	$38,175 – $136,237
Health Services Administration	$37,050 – $161,400
Health Education/Behavioral Science	$33,000 – $86,625
Environmental Health	$44,550 – $143,700
International Health	$31,500 – $86,625
Nutrition	$31,500 – $70,875
Public Health Practice/Program Management	$41,175 – $102,000
Biomedical Laboratory	$31,500 – $78,750

Planning a Program of Study

Choosing a Major

There is no single recommended undergraduate major for students intending to apply to a school of public health. Students of public health come from a variety of educational backgrounds; a quality undergraduate education is a plus for any applicant.

However, there are some undergraduate majors that can be beneficial when applying to a school of public health. For example, to study Epidemiology or Biostatistics, a major in math or basic science is ideal. For an education in Behavioral Sciences or Health Education, consider sociology, psychology or anthropology as a major. For studying Health Services Administration, consider a business or political science background. To study Global Health, a social science degree is helpful. For those who want to study Environmental Health, consider studying either biology or chemistry. Maternal and Child Health lends itself to both biology and social sciences.

Acquiring public health experience

Most schools do accept students without prior work experience; however, all schools look favorably on applicants who have at least a little experience, so students should consider pursuing some experience before applying to schools of public health. It is also suggested that applicants contact the schools that they are most interested in attending to ask about their specific requirements.

There are many options for individuals who are looking to gain experience before applying to a school of public health. Examples are:

- Working part-time or full-time at a hospital or health clinic, such as working on an immunization program, a reproductive health clinic or a health promotion program.
- Volunteering for a non-profit direct services organization such as a Community Health Center, an HIV/AIDS clinic or a local chapter of the Red Cross.
- Working at a non-profit organization that is directly involved in public health advocacy and policy, either in the US or abroad.
- Working or volunteering for a local health department.

Schools recognize that it is sometimes difficult to gain experience before applying, so some schools of public health have developed programs that offer opportunities for potential applicants to get experience before applying.

Prospective students may also conduct informational interviews with members of the public health community. Many schools look upon this experience as providing at least some exposure to public health, which is helpful in the application process.

The Admissions Process

While schools of public health look for high graduate entrance exam scores and GPA, other aspects of an applicant's record, such as career achievement, professional experience, and clarity of career goals, are equally important. Admissions decisions are based on an overall assessment of the ability of applicants to successfully complete the degree track area selected. Each program or track within a given department may set additional requirements for admission; therefore, applicants should refer to the individual programs for details. All schools of public health require effective verbal and written communication; therefore, students should try to take advantage of undergraduate opportunities to hone these skills.

A typical application package would include:
- Completed application and fee (some institutions may require an application to both the graduate school and an addendum for the specific MPH program).
- A personal statement describing the student's interest in and potential for contributing to the field of public health.
- A resume reflecting work/volunteer history.
- Evidence of an earned baccalaureate or graduate degree or equivalent from an accredited institution of higher education.
- Official transcripts of all academic work.
- A strong undergraduate record overall, with a grade point average of 3.0 or better in the subject of the major.
- Three letters of recommendation from academic or professional references.
- Submission of one standardized test (e.g. GRE, MCAT, GMAT) scores within the last five years. Some institutions may allow for substitution of DAT or LSAT.

In 2006, the schools of public health launched a centralized application service, SOPHAS. As of this publication date, 22 out of the 38 CEPH-accredited schools of public health are participating in this service and several more are anticipated to participate in the application year 2007-2008.

SOPHAS is open from approximately the beginning of September through early-mid August of each year. Applicants will need to provide original transcripts to SOPHAS, three recommendations, a personal essay for each designated school and test scores as may be required by individual schools of public health. Applicants can also upload a CV or resume, and submit their work, research and service history in the application.

Schools of public health have multiple deadlines, so applicants are asked to keep a close eye on the list of deadlines found on the SOPHAS.ORG website. Once the application has been e-submitted, applicants can monitor the progress of their application and their submitted documents.

Instructions, customer service contact information and a complete check-list of items need to complete the application can be found at www.sophas.org.

Financing Your Education

In 2004-2005, the average yearly cost of a master's level degree in public health, including tuition, fees, books, etc. was $18,665 and the median was just over $18,035. The range is from $3,665 to $33,225 per year. Most master's programs are two years in length. However, there are also accelerated programs, distance learning programs, programs for part-time students, etc.

Students may wish to defray these expenses through the wide variety of assistance programs that are available to public health students, such as scholarships, grants, loans, and work programs. Students should contact the school they will be attending and ask about university-based student aid programs. Many schools have endowments for student aid for which matriculating students would be eligible.

Students who are willing to pursue their degree part-time are encouraged to ask about their school's tuition remission programs. Many colleges subsidize or pay full tuition for employees that enroll in courses. These types of programs are useful in reducing reliance on student loan programs; however, students must balance that benefit against the additional time it will take to complete their degree program on a part-time basis.

The National Health Service Corps (NHSC) offers tuition assistance and living stipends for students participating in some Public Health disciplines in exchange for service in a federally-mandated health manpower shortage area after leaving school. More information about this program is available at nhsc.bhpr.hrsa.gov or by calling (800) 638-0824.

Public health students are encouraged to investigate scholarship and financial aid programs such as www.fastweb.com, www.finaid.org, www.fafsa.org and studentaid.ed.gov/PORTALSWebApp/students/english/index.jsp.

Public Health Credentialing

An independent organization called the National Board of Public Health Examiners is currently developing a credential for graduates of CEPH-accredited schools of public health and MPH programs. The credential shall be conferred to graduates who successfully pass the NBPHE exam, which will first be administered in the summer 2008. It is likely that someday soon, this exam will be considered the gold standard for graduates in public health. More information can be found at: www.nbphe.org.

Resources

Association of Schools of Public Health, www.asph.org

Association of Schools of Public Health
1101 15th Street NW Suite 910
Washington DC 20005
(202) 296-1099
fax: (202) 296-1252
info@asph.org
www.asph.org

www.whatispublichealth.org

VETERINARY MEDICINE (D.V.M.)

General Description

Traditionally, veterinarians have maintained healthy and productive commercial food animals and livestock, secured public health, and treated illness and disease in livestock, and sport and companion animals. Today, however, the breadth of veterinary medicine encompasses much more. The majority of veterinarians are in private small, large or mixed animal clinical practice; however, county, state and federal governments, universities, private industry, zoos, the U.S. military, wildlife organizations, racetracks, and circuses are also some of the diverse settings that employ veterinarians.

About 75% of the approximately 85,000 veterinarians in the United States work in private practice. During the past twenty years, the nature of private practice has evolved to cater to increasing demands by animal owners and production animal managers. No longer are practices focused only on large animals in the classical rural large animal or equine practice, or to dogs and cats in a suburban neighborhood small animal practice. Many large animal practitioners now consult on herd-health issues, with some traveling great distances to deliver their expertise. Emergency animal clinics service trauma victims much as do trauma centers in urban hospitals. Board Certified Specialists run referral practices in specialty fields such as critical care, dentistry, dermatology, internal medicine, ophthalmology, radiology and surgery. Mobile veterinary services come to your home, and mobile surgeons contract with general practitioners in their offices. Practices limited to dogs, cats, avian medicine, exotic animals (reptiles, amphibians, etc.), aquatic animals, cancer treatment, low-cost spaying-neutering, in vitro fertilization, geriatric care, preventive medicine (acupuncture, nutrition, etc.), and in-home euthanasia, all exist. And there are bound to be more changes in future types of practices developed due to increased specialization and to competition in the veterinary marketplace. The other 25% of veterinarians work for county and state governments, private industry, U.S. military, universities, humane associations, and other organizations.

The following federal agencies employ a large number of veterinarians: U.S. Department of Agriculture, Food and Drug Administration, National Institutes of Health Centers for Disease Control and Prevention, Department of Defense, and the U.S. Fish and Wildlife Service. Veterinarians employed by government entities enforce regulations established to protect public health and the health of animals (domestic and wild), eradicate diseases such as rabies and brucellosis, and ensure the quality, safety and wholesomeness of foods and animal-derived products. Universities and industry employ veterinarians to conduct basic and advance biomedical research with laboratory animals. Their goal is to better understand disease processes and develop methods for their control or cure in both animals and humans. Biomedical research continually produces major advances in pharmaceuticals and disease treatments. Veterinarians are also educators in universities. This list is far from complete. See your health professions advisor to discuss these and other possible veterinary careers, which may be of interest to you.

You may be interested in an area closely related to veterinary medicine that does not require a veterinary degree. Such areas include animal welfare, animal training and breeding, hospital administration, wildlife conservation, marine biology, agriculture, etc. The American Veterinary Medical Association (AVMA) Directory, published annually, lists national and international organizations associated with these activities and their addresses so you may contact them concerning additional career possibilities. Contact the AVMA for information about the AVMA Directory (see Resources) or an AVMA member veterinarian.

The Decision to Pursue a Career in Veterinary Medicine

"I have always wanted to be a veterinarian." Most veterinarians will tell you that their interest in animals and animal health began when they were very young. Perhaps the spark was lit by experiences with a beloved family pet, toiling on a farm, riding horses, visiting a zoo, or walks through the woods. For others, the spark was lit later in life and may have focused on research, public health, animal welfare, or ecological issues. People come to veterinary medicine from all types of backgrounds with diverse goals. Many enter the profession when they are young, while others may gain their degree after a successful career in another field. A number of students enter a veterinary college with an advanced degree such as an M.S. or Ph.D. Others have yet to graduate from an undergraduate college.

Whatever your background and motivation, you have decided that you wish to prepare for a veterinary medical education. With a degree in veterinary medicine, your options for professional success and fulfillment are broad. This section will give you appropriate information for charting your course and setting realistic goals for yourself.

Outlook for the Future in Veterinary Medicine

The outlook for veterinary medicine, in companion and production animal practice, along with research and public practice, remains bright. The profession continues to see growth, especially in government, research, and other forms of public practice. Numerous opportunities lie outside of standard clinical practice. This is especially evident in response to the threat of bioterrorism and national security needs. At present, there is a shortage of veterinarians who enter research and public practice as a whole. Those interested in public practice and research have many open doors. Veterinarians are also being called upon to work on issues pertinent to the environment, conservation, aquaculture, wildlife management, and overall ecological health.

Opportunities and employment for veterinarians in companion animal practice, including horses, are expected to continue to grow. While the number of pets is expected to remain stable, rising incomes and the maturation of the boomers are expected to fuel the demand for high-quality companion animal care. More veterinary services are now available due to increased specialization and medical technology. There are more effective treatment modalities for acute and chronic problems and veterinary practices are becoming more flexible. More pet owners are also taking advantage of non-traditional veterinary services, including acupuncture, holistic medicine, physical therapy, behavior consultation, prophylactic dentistry, etc. With the advent of new and specialized procedures and medicines, pet owners may be willing to pay more for elective and intensive care than in the past. Pet owners are even purchasing pet insurance, increasing the likelihood that a considerable amount of money will be spent on veterinary care for their pets. The level of income of companion animal practitioners has increased in recent years and reflects the current and projected shifts in the supply and demand of veterinarians. As with most healthcare professions, practitioner salaries reflect regional demand and level of urbanization.

Food animal veterinarians have seen dramatic changes the nature of their practices over the past decades. The number of farms with animals in the U.S. has dropped precipitously, while the number of animals per farm has increased. Whereas in 1980 there were 334,000 farms with at least one dairy cow and an average of 32 head, the year 2002 saw only 92,000 farms, but an average of 99 head. This type of consolidation is seen in cattle, poultry and swine production as well. These dramatic changes were the result of a combination of low commodities prices, higher feed costs, and competition. The veterinarian's role focuses less on the individual animal and more on the health of the herd. Demand for veterinarians with specialized knowledge in herd-health issues is very strong and these individuals command high salaries.

Demand for specialists, in many areas, including ophthalmology, internal medicine, toxicology, laboratory animal medicine, etc. is expected to continue to increase. Many students, during their third year of veterinary school, consider further education through internships as a lead-in to a residency program. Internships and residencies are optional and not required to become a licensed, practicing veterinarian.

Planning a Program of Study

The veterinary medical profession is much smaller than human medicine. While there are 130 allopathic medical colleges, there are only 28 colleges and schools of veterinary medicine in the U.S. There is no distinction between a college and a school of veterinary medicine and the terms will be used interchangeably throughout the chapter. In 2005, there were 2,645 positions available for first-year students and over 4,500 applicants applied through the central application service, Veterinary Medical College Application Service (VMCAS) administered by the Association of American Veterinary Medical Colleges. Others applied directly to select individual schools. The number of seats available is not expected to significantly rise in the near future. The number of underrepresented students in Veterinary Medicine such as, African American, Hispanic, Native American and Asian applicants was 10% of the total applicant enrollment of veterinarian students in 2005.

The number of women applying and matriculating into veterinary school has changed the face of veterinary medicine profoundly, and is now nearly 80% of all veterinary students. The increase in the number of female applicants and enrolled students mirrors a less dramatic increase in women entering other professional medical fields.

In response to the changing applicant pool and national needs for veterinarians, veterinary medical schools have changed or are considering changing some of their admission practices. Many now actively recruit students by making high school and college visitations, as well as by offering special admission and summer enrichment programs for disadvantaged students. Combined DVM/VMD ,Ph.D., MPH, and MBA programs are increasing in numbers. Colleges may recruit applicants, especially those with research interests, into one of these programs. While recruitment efforts may be increasing, the number of graduates has remained relatively constant over the past 20 years. The number of accredited veterinary colleges has increased by one since 1983, with the Western University of Health Sciences College of Veterinary Medicine admitting its first class in 2003.

Many individuals desire to enter the profession and practice medicine or pursue related interests. The individual colleges set their own admission criteria and have the sole discretion concerning student admissions. Not every qualified applicant will be accepted. Thus, part of your professional plan should consist of options should you not be accepted to a veterinary college. It is imperative that you keep your options open. Should you not gain admission and remain committed to becoming a veterinarian, do not become discouraged. You are not alone. Many students gain admission their second application cycle. Consult with your advisor — where there is a will, there usually is a way.

As with any aspect of life, having a plan to achieve a goal is essential. Your goal is to gain admission to a college of veterinary medicine and create your path to professional success. Many considerations, including academics, experience, debt load, program of study, family life and more need to be taken into account when planning your professional path. The following sections explain the requirements and steps necessary to make yourself a competitive candidate for admission into a college of veterinary medicine. A wealth of information sources exist concerning veterinary applications, colleges and careers. Use them well.

The term "preprofessional requirements" defines the characteristics and requirements necessary to submit a complete application to a college of veterinary medicine. Successful completion of your preprofessional requirements includes finishing all required coursework, maintenance of a high GPA, scoring well on required standardized exams, gaining exposure to different aspects of veterinary medicine, and taking on leadership roles in activities on campus or in the community. Applicants who are deficient in any of the above are at a disadvantage, compared to other applicants. Each of the above will be discussed in detail below.

Required Coursework

Each college or school of veterinary medicine has its own list of required courses to be completed prior to matriculation. (Some schools require that prerequisite courses be completed during the fall semester prior to matriculation; some require spring semester completion; and some allow completion of prerequisite courses during the summer semester immediately prior to matriculation.) Admission will be denied if said courses are not completed on time. Most colleges require that all of your science and math courses be taken within the past 4–10 years. Below is a summary of courses required by many of the colleges and schools. Not all of the courses are required for each school. You may be fortunate in attending an undergraduate college that offers all of the courses required for the schools to which you plan to submit an application. If there is a course not offered by your undergraduate college, consult with the veterinary colleges to determine if another closely-related course can be substituted. This is a common occurrence with animal science courses. If no substitution can be made, you may need to consider other options, such as taking the course at a different undergraduate college (possibly during the summer), inquire if the course can be taken via a distance-learning or web-based class, or transfer to another undergraduate college. Consult the *Veterinary Medical School Admissions Requirements (VMSAR)* book, your advisor or the college to learn about the college's specific requirements. Requirements do change, so you should check annually to see if there are any changes, which may impact your academic plan.

Math and Sciences

Algebra /Trigonometry	Calculus / Precalculus
Animal sciences	Animal nutrition
Biology with lab	Cell biology
Inorganic Chemistry with lab	Organic Chemistry with lab
General Physics	Biochemistry
Embryology	Genetics
Microbiology	Statistics
Zoology	Immunology

Non-Sciences

English Composition	Literature
Humanities/Arts and	Public Speaking/Speech
Social Sciences	Behavioral Sciences

A few schools require business/finance, physiology, vertebrate anatomy, technical writing, history, economics, computer skills course.

1. **Math**

   If you have a weak math background or it has been a long time since you have taken math, consider taking an introductory or intermediate algebra class to prepare for upper-level math. It is important that your mathematics abilities are strong. Even if calculus is not required by your colleges of interest, analytical skills are critical to your success in chemistry, physics, statistics, and computer science.

2. **Chemistry**

Most students agree — chemistry is difficult to master. If your chemistry background is weak, consider taking an introductory course. Some undergraduate colleges give placement exams in their beginning-level general chemistry course. Discuss the results with your preveterinary advisor or instructor. Be mindful that many students struggle with chemistry courses. Most of the schools currently require at least one course in biochemistry, which means you will be taking a sequence of two to three years of chemistry courses (inorganic, organic and biochemistry). Give yourself every advantage by building a good foundation in the beginning. Remember, the later you begin your chemistry sequence, the longer it will be before you may apply to veterinary school.

3. **Other Sciences**

All veterinary colleges require one or more semesters of physics and biology, and many require genetics, microbiology, biochemistry, nutrition or other upper division biology courses such as embryology or immunology.

4. **English, Humanities, Social Sciences and Behavioral Sciences**

The majority of veterinary schools require courses in both English and humanities, and most undergraduate institutions include varying amounts of these in graduation requirements. Several veterinary schools require courses in social sciences, business, and public speaking. In addition, all of the standardized examinations include an analysis of reading ability.

Choice of Major

The veterinary profession is broad and wide-ranging. Colleges and schools of veterinary medicine seek applicants with diverse educational backgrounds. English majors have gained admission, as have those who have majored in a variety of other fields. However, schools generally select students who have strong backgrounds in the sciences. It is important that you choose a field that interests you, but enables you to complete all of the required courses (see above). Thus, it is not essential that you have a major in a science. If you are required to take the Biology Subject GRE test, a major in Biology will prepare you for that test better than any other major.

The Admission Process

Completing your applications to veterinary colleges can be a daunting task. Each college has its own academic, examination and experience requirements, expectations and deadlines. Many also have specific application requirements. However, the schools all put emphasis on the following criteria as they review candidates.

Factors evaluated by Admissions Committees

1. **Academic Record**

Although veterinary admissions committees evaluate many criteria when selecting a veterinary class, academic performance remains one of the most important factors in the committees' decisions as they are seeking evidence that you will be able to successfully complete the rigorous DVM program. If you are like most preveterinary students, you want to understand the role of your grades in the admission process. Here is a typical statement from a veterinary school catalog, "Demonstration of outstanding academic achievement is a necessary prerequisite for admission to the professional veterinary medical curriculum." How to define "outstanding academic achievement," of course, is quite another question. You will be able to glean information from *VMSAR* or the college's website. These sources contain the average GPAs and test scores from the previously admitted class.

Method of application evaluation and weight placed on various admissions criteria varies from school to school. Many schools have a point system, which gives weight to various criteria, while a few schools now use a subjective evaluation process which allows for a broad, overall evaluation of the application. In a typical admission process, academic factors count for about 50% of your score or ranking. Generally, equal weight is given to the undergraduate cumulative GPA, GPA for the last year or two of undergraduate work, GPA for the required science courses and finally, the standardized test. The other 50% of your evaluation may be based on "non-academic" factors, which will vary from school to school. It is important to be aware of the evaluation criteria and processes for the schools to which you are applying.

Most schools require that all preveterinary courses be taken for a letter grade, as admission committee members wish to see what level you achieved and evaluate all applicants equally. Therefore you place yourself a disadvantage if you take these courses pass/fail or if you attend an undergraduate institution that does not assign grades. Each veterinary school has its own policy for course repeats and GPA calculations. Some schools include repeats in the GPA calculation, some do not. If you received a low grade and it was due to factors other than your study skills and the college does not require repeating the course, then improving your performance in a more difficult course should compensate. If you did not really master the material and other courses build on it, you should probably repeat the course. However, several low grades in required courses may mean your strategy or your goals are inappropriate. Your preveterinary advisor will be able to counsel you on how to proceed. Also admissions committees often view inordinate numbers of withdrawals on a transcript to be a sign of the applicant's inability to master the material, despite the final grade in the course.

While overall GPA is important, the colleges pay special attention to applicants' science-based or math/science-based GPA. Even if the overall GPA is high, a low science GPA will disadvantage an applicant. Many colleges have a minimum acceptable science GPA (see *VMSAR*). Geographical boundaries may place an added requirement on students: schools tend to have higher overall GPA requirements for out-of-state at-large applicants. A student who takes an average or greater number of units per semester, has a GPA in the range of 3.4 to 3.8 or better and has excellent non-academic factors (discussed below) will be an outstanding candidate. Remember, grades account for a significant portion of the weight of your application. Be mindful that a 4.0 is not a free ticket into veterinary school. The remainder of your application must be outstanding, as well. And yes, students with a 4.0 have been denied admission in the past.

2. **Standardized Examinations**

   All of the colleges require scores from at least one examination. Currently, there are three different examinations utilized: The Graduate Record Examination (GRE), Medical College Admission Test (MCAT) or GRE Biology Subject test. The greatest number of veterinary colleges and schools require or accept scores from the GRE general test. The Veterinary College Admission Test (VCAT) has been discontinued. Contact individual colleges regarding their acceptance of old VCAT scores. Acceptance of particular examinations varies by college. Most require or accept the GRE General test, but a few require either the MCAT or Biology Subject test. Thus, it is important that you identify which exam(s) you will take and when it will be appropriate to take them. Deadlines for receipt of test scores vary by school. For testing dates and information, see the websites of the test administering organizations (Resources). The colleges have limits as to the oldest scores they will accept. This ranges from two to six years.

   There are no specific college courses to help prepare you for the General GRE test other than mathematics through college algebra, trigonometry and introductory English. Therefore, it may be to your advantage to prepare for and take the GRE early, perhaps after your second year in college. Most applicants take the exam in the spring of the year when they are applying to veterinary school. Consult the GRE Bulletin or website for test centers and dates. When selecting a date to take the exam, be sure to allow enough preparation time before the exam, and leave yourself enough time to receive your scores from the first attempt and to strengthen your knowledge in any weak areas, so that you can improve your scores if you need to retake it.

   The GRE Biology Subject Test is designed for students majoring in biology. Not only should students have completed an introductory year biology course, but also many students report that some advanced courses in subjects such as genetics and ecology are especially helpful to their preparation. There are, naturally, many courses that can be added to this list, but you should discuss your strengths and weaknesses with your advisor before planning. Thus, plan to take the Biology Subject test no later than the spring prior to submitting your application so you have time to retake it, if necessary.

3. **Animal and Health-Related Experience**

   While academics play a significant role in the admissions process, most competitive candidates have similar GPAs and standardized test scores. Experiences and employment history can help distinguish applicants from each other. Animal and health-related experiences may account for up to one-third of the weight of an application. Admission committees utilize an applicant's experiences to:

   - Demonstrate an applicant's sincere interest in veterinary medicine and the biological sciences.

   - Show that an applicant has developed a realistic and accurate understanding of the veterinary medical profession. Besides the immediately obvious benefits of acquiring such a familiarity with the profession, this becomes important when an applicant is asked to discuss his/her understanding of the veterinary medical profession in the narrative portion of the application and in the interview.

   - Define and reaffirm the applicant's desire to enter the veterinary profession and to formulate his/her future goals and objectives. This is where interest in non-traditional career goals can be demonstrated.

   - Show that the student has a sense of confidence and comfort around a variety of animals, which is essential in handling the animals that one will encounter throughout the curriculum.

   Developing breadth of experience in different veterinary settings, such as a combination of small, large and exotic animal veterinary work and research is to your advantage. Students should make every effort to acquire a basic understanding of the veterinary medical profession as a whole. Non-veterinary experiences include areas where you work with animals but are not directly supervised by a veterinarian, such as on a farm; training horses, grooming dogs and cats; at the local zoo; pet adoption programs, pet therapy, or animal shelters; and non-animal related, such as in a chemistry or computer laboratory. Other positions, non-animal related, may show other special skills or abilities that you have. The positions that you work may be formal or informal, paid, unpaid or volunteer. It is important to demonstrate that you are well-rounded and can adapt to a variety of roles. Most schools require a minimum number of hours of animal and veterinary medicine exposure. It is always a good idea to have above the minimum in order to demonstrate a high level of motivation and extensive experience.

   All veterinary school applicants are requested to provide certain facts on the application about veterinary and animal/health-related experiences, including number of hours worked, inclusive dates, responsibilities and names of supervisors and advisors. If you keep accurate records of this information while obtaining the experience, you will find it much easier to completely and accurately fill out this part of the application. Plan ahead.

   There are many ways to acquire experience, including:

   - **Internship Programs.** Your campus career planning and placement office, biology, animal sciences, biochemistry, microbiology, etc. departments or preveterinary advisor may provide a list of internships where you can work on or off campus in veterinary practices, zoos, institutions, organizations, etc. Internships are usually on a volunteer basis, although some paid positions occasionally become available. Some internships may be taken for college credit.

- **Private Veterinary Practices.** Obtaining experience in a private practice may involve offering your services on a voluntary basis to a practicing veterinarian, but more frequently, paid positions can be arranged. This experience may vary from simply observing the veterinarian in surgery to actively participating in many aspects of day-to-day private practice. In any case, this will probably be the most important type of experience that you will obtain since it offers enormous potential for you to learn about the intricacies of the veterinary profession. Many students begin in a small animal or mixed animal practice.

- **Research.** Independent study programs in any area of the health sciences may be pursued by a motivated upper-division student. You must generally connect with a faculty advisor who will support your project in his/her research laboratory. Although research experience is not required by the veterinary schools, it provides a way in which you can use the knowledge you have acquired in a problem-solving environment. There are many places to consider for research experience both during the academic year and during the summer. Feel free to pursue any type of scientific research that interests you.

- **Special Resources.** Some undergraduate colleges are associated with veterinary schools that have primate centers, raptor centers, or commercial animal programs; some cities have large aquatic parks, wild animal parks, and zoos; and you may be able to work for a private wildlife organization or a government agency such as the U.S. Fish and Wildlife Service during the summer.

- **Enrichment Programs.** Several veterinary schools have summer enrichment programs to help minority and disadvantaged students prepare for and gain admission to veterinary school. These programs can help to upgrade your academic and noncognitive qualifications. Contact your preveterinary advisor or the schools individually. The *VMSAR* also has a list of these programs.

- **Other possibilities for obtaining experience do exist.** Use your imagination. Do not be afraid to knock on doors and sell yourself. Have you heard of horseback riding programs for people with physical-impairments? How about helping to hatch penguins at Sea World? Talk to students in your local preveterinary club. They may exchange information about positions with veterinarians. Of course, you will want to find out about opportunities in your own area.

4. **Letters of evaluation**

Letters of evaluation are required by veterinary schools, and are utilized as another source of information to demonstrate your special qualities and interests. Personal letters of recommendation provide the admissions committees with information which cannot be assessed by grades or academic performance alone. They showcase your personality, interests and drive to succeed. More information is provided about letters of evaluation in chapter 2.

5. **Leadership and Communication Skills**

Are you a leader or a follower? Are you a team player and get along well with others? It is of benefit to students if they have been able to demonstrate leadership qualities and strong communication skills. Holding offices on campus, such as on the student health advisory board or in the preveterinary club can be beneficial. There are many community organizations as well that afford you the opportunity for leadership experience. Skills can also be demonstrated through work experience, student government, teaching assistantships, youth mentoring, etc. Veterinarians are leaders in their practices, in the community, and in many medical and public health fields and the veterinary schools look to applicants for future leadership.

6. **Commitment to Service**

Veterinary schools are looking for individuals who show compassion and are interested in giving back to the community. Therefore, involvement in volunteer service is an important learning experience. Many campuses have student volunteer programs, or look around in your community for opportunities. You can get involved in volunteer service of any kind that interests you.

7. **The Interview**

Some veterinary schools require an interview; some only interview some portion of their acceptable applicant pool; others do not interview at all. Be prepared for the interview format and review the material in chapter 2. Interviews are unique experiences for most applicants. They are another opportunity to demonstrate your personal qualities and accomplishments and most importantly to convey your understanding of and motivation for the veterinary profession.

The Application

1. **When and where to apply**

Apply when you are prepared to present yourself as a qualified applicant. In the early spring of the year you plan to apply to veterinary school, begin to prepare your application materials. Most students who want to go directly to vet school after college begin their application during the spring of their junior (third) year of their undergraduate education and submit the application in the fall of their senior year. Very well-qualified students who can complete the required coursework and credit hours, experiences and tests, may submit their application in the fall of their second or third year. A smaller number of individuals are accepted from the pool of second and third-year applicants than from the pool of those who submit their application during the fall of their senior year. This is due to the fact that younger students have not had time to acquire adequate work and life experiences. You can gain practice and experience by submitting an application, but keep in mind that it is better to submit your best application the first time.

a. **Timeline for applying**

Applications are normally available early in the summer. Applicants spend the summer months preparing the application, seeking evaluators for the required letters of recommendation, and gathering transcripts. Most applications are due October 1; all are due in the early fall. Verify with each school the specific application deadlines for that school.

b. **Selecting Schools or Colleges of Interest**

In order to begin selecting schools where you will apply, there are many factors to consider: geographic location, residency requirements, personal support system (presence of family or friends), cost and financial aid, curriculum, special programs, facilities, support for disadvantaged students, preveterinary course requirements and type of admission examination required. Most students look at three or four colleges or schools of veterinary medicine, but there is no limit. It is to your advantage to educate yourself as much as possible about all of these factors.

c. **Residency Considerations and Contracts**

Geographic boundaries, such as your state or country of residence, used to limit an applicant's choice of veterinary colleges. However, many veterinary colleges, public and private, are enrolling many more non-residents. This is a shift and is to the applicant's advantage. Although all colleges accept non-residents, there are many fewer seats for non-residents than residents. Some colleges accept out-of-state students and allow them to become residents and pay resident tuition after one year.

Most states without a veterinary college contract with one or more colleges of veterinary medicine to enroll a certain number of students from the contracting state. A specific number of seats are allotted to the state but contracts with the veterinary schools frequently change. The *VMSAR* book contains a section outlining all of the contracts available as of press time. It is best to consult the *VMSAR* book annually. Many of the contracts are only financial in nature and do not give preference to the applicant over other non-residents. You may apply to all of the colleges that contract with your state or any other college based on your strengths and perception of your chances for admission. Your advisor may have suggestions regarding contract seats. Also, be aware of residency requirements in each state, i.e. you must live in the state for so many years or months as a non-student, have a state driver's license, pay taxes, etc. You may need to be certified as a contract student during your application process. If so, it is your responsibility to register with your state.

If you live in a state without a veterinary college it is wise to be aware of your options at several colleges outside of your state and to apply to more than one college. In the past, an applicant usually submitted one or two applications. With the advent of a centralized application service and increased acceptance of non-residents, the average number of applications submitted through the centralized application service is between three and four. Submitting more than two applications has traditionally been a strategy of many students as the success of applicants submitting three or more applications is substantially higher than for those submitting two or fewer.

2. **Veterinary Medical College Application Service**
Most of the colleges utilize the centralized application service through the Veterinary Medical College Application Service (VMCAS). VMCAS is sponsored by the Association of American Veterinary Medical Colleges (AAVMC) in Washington, DC. The application is web-based and is completed by the applicant only once per admission cycle. VMCAS distributes the application to the colleges designated by the applicant.

The web-based application becomes available for students in late May/early June and may be found through the AAVMC's website (www.aavmc.org). The application can be completed at the applicant's discretion, over several months. Your personal statement and evaluations are also completed through VMCAS.

The VMCAS website contains valuable information concerning completion of the application as well as general information on the application process. Even with a centralized application, applying is quite time consuming. VMCAS saves the applicant the work of completing multiple application forms when she/he is applying to multiple schools. Some colleges prefer to utilize their own applications and do not participate in VMCAS. Others utilize the service for out-of-state applicants only. The VMCAS website details level of participation for each college. Also, many colleges require completion of supplemental application forms. Your application will not be considered if you do not also submit the supplemental application. Check the colleges' websites for specific information on submitting a supplemental application.

VMCAS maintains a staff to address questions or problems with the VMCAS process itself but all questions pertaining to specific policies of the participating schools must be directed to the schools themselves. The VMCAS website provides links to the individual colleges for your convenience. You must request applications individually from each school that does not participate in VMCAS. The applications are usually available in late May or June.

An important part of your application will be the personal statement that you will write. It is your opportunity to give the admissions committee a look into your life, aspirations and unique attributes. The committees also utilize the personal statement to assess your writing and communications skills. It usually requires you to discuss (a) the events that led you to choose veterinary medicine as a career, (b) how your background and personal interests relate to the desire to become a veterinarian, (c) your understanding of veterinary medicine as a profession and (d) your career goals and objectives. Committees are also interested in what unique qualities you will bring to the class and to the profession. Be certain to answer these questions in a well-organized, complete, and professional manner. This is especially true in supplemental application narratives. The admission committee will use this narrative in an attempt to understand the quality of animal and veterinary experiences gained by the applicant. Students should, therefore, use the narrative to convey what they have learned about the veterinary profession, not merely what they have experienced as a part of it. Avoid negative or pessimistic connotations or undertones. A well-written narrative will, instead, present you as an optimistic, positive individual. Lastly, the narrative should be unique and interesting, as well as grammatically correct and error free.

The VMCAS application also requires that you enter the names and contact information for three evaluators through its Electronic Letters of Recommendation system (eLOR). All of the schools your VMCAS application is delivered to will contain these three electronic letters. If applying through VMCAS, you cannot have evaluators tailor letters to specific colleges, unless you are applying only to one college. Once you enter the evaluators' names into the VMCAS application, the evaluators will be able to complete their evaluations online, saving applicants from worrying about letters becoming lost in the mail or misplaced. The system also allows applicants to check if their evaluations have been submitted. Should your evaluator not desire to submit information online, he or she may send in a paper form. However, you should provide him or her with the form. The form can be downloaded from the VMCAS website. Be mindful that two colleges ONLY accept letters electronically and most colleges will soon follow this practice. It is recommended that you have all of your VMCAS evaluations submitted electronically. The applicant is responsible for ensuring the timely submission of their three evaluations. Some schools may request additional letters beyond these three. You should follow the same procedure and send all letters to VMCAS. VMCAS will then forward them to your colleges. As mentioned however, evaluations can not be tailor made for specific colleges. All evaluations will be sent directly to all your designated colleges. Colleges not participating in VMCAS have their own evaluation submission policies and require evaluations be sent directly to them.

Resources

Veterinary Medical Associations:
> Association of American Veterinary Medical Colleges (www.aavmc.org)
> American Veterinary Medical Association (www.avma.org)
> For a complete list of the 28 US veterinary schools, visit www.avma.org.

Veterinary Medical School Admissions Requirements published annually by the AAVMC. See www.aavmc.org for ordering information.

Services for evaluations of transcripts from foreign colleges:
> Joseph Silney and Associates, Inc. (www.jsilney.com)
> World Education Service (www.wes.org)
> American Association of Collegiate and Registrars and Admissions Officers (www.aacrao.org)

APPENDIX A
CAREER SUMMARIES

ALLOPATHIC PHYSICIAN (M.D.)

Summarized from the *U.S. Bureau of Labor Statistics Occupational Outlook Handbook 2008-2009*. For a complete description, see **www.bls.gov/oco/ocos074.htm**.

I. *Career Description*

Physicians are licensed practitioners who perform medical examinations, diagnose illnesses, treat people who are suffering from disease or injury and advise patients on maintaining good health. They may be general practitioners or specialists. There are twenty-four specialty boards (or areas); the largest medical specialties for which there is graduate training include internal medicine, family medicine, general surgery, obstetrics and gynecology, psychiatry, pediatrics, radiology, anesthesiology, ophthalmology, pathology, and orthopedic surgery. Some physicians combine the practice of medicine with research and/or teaching in medical schools, i.e., academic medicine.

II. *Career Settings*

Most physicians are in private practices, in group practices, or salaried employees of managed care organizations. The number and size of group practices are growing, probably as a response to the high cost of technological equipment and malpractice insurance. Physicians practice in a great variety of settings, including hospitals and clinics, Health Maintenance Organizations (HMOs), surgicenters, public health agencies, research laboratories, nursing homes, military medical facilities, business firms, schools, and prisons.

III. *Compensation*

(Represents median total compensation for allopathic and osteopathic physicians over one year in the specialty in 2005)

Internal Medicine Physicians $166,420
Surgeons $282,504
Anesthesiologists $321,686
Pediatricians $161,331
Family Practitioners $156,010
Obstetrics/Gynecology $247,348

IV. *Educational Requirements for Practice*

Undergraduate Education: All medical schools require at least the equivalent of three years of college; many require a baccalaureate degree. Most students enter medical school with at least a bachelor's degree, and many have advanced degrees.

Professional School: 4-year professional degree program in a School or College of Medicine.

Graduate Medical Education: 3-8 years of residency and/or fellowship training. Physicians who wish to teach and/or conduct research may also earn a Ph.D. degree.

V. Licensing

All states require physicians to be licensed. In order to obtain a license, the applicant must graduate from an accredited school of medicine and successfully complete the United States Medical Licensing Examination (USMLE), steps 1, 2, and 3. Administration of a clinical skills examination, Step 2 Clinical Skills, began in June 2004. In addition, most states require one or two years of supervised residency in an accredited graduate medical education program. The Board of Examiners in each state can supply specific information regarding licensure.

VI. Resources

American Medical Association (AMA)
515 North State Street
Chicago, IL 60610
800/621-8335
www.ama-assn.org

Association of American Medical Colleges (AAMC)
2450 N Street NW
Washington, DC 20037
202/828-0400
www.aamc.org

CHIROPRACTOR (D.C.)

Summarized from the *U.S. Bureau of Labor Statistics Occupational Outlook Handbook 2008-2009*. For a complete description, see **www.bls.gov/oco/ocos071.htm**.

I. Career Description

Doctors of Chiropractic are health care providers who practice through non-drug, non-surgical means. They believe that the relationship between the structure and function of the human body is significant. Chiropractors postulate that spinal manipulation by way of chiropractic adjustments will correct disturbances of the nervous system caused by derangement of the musculoskeletal structure. Therapies used in conjunction with spinal manipulation include physiotherapy, acupuncture, and nutrition. Diagnostic techniques include the taking of patient history, routine exams, x-ray and lab tests.

II. Career Settings

Chiropractors typically work in private offices, clinics and chiropractic hospitals.

III. Compensation

The median annual income in 2006 was $65,220 per year. The middle 50 percent earned between $45,710 and $96,500 a year. (*Occupational Outlook Handbook 2008-2009*)

IV. Educational Requirements for Practice

Undergraduate Education: Chiropractic requires a minimum of two years of preprofessional education. Many students have a bachelor's degree.

Professional School: 3-4 year professional degree program in a School or College of Chiropractic Medicine.

V. Licensing

To gain licensure, students must complete their professional schooling of four years and pass both the basic science and chiropractic sections of the National Board of Chiropractic Examiners. All states administer a state board exam following the passing of the national exam. No internship or residency is required for practice.

VI. Resources

Council on Chiropractic Education (CCE)
8049 North 85th Way
Scottsdale, AZ 85258
480/443-8877
www.cce-usa.org

American Chiropractic Association
1701 Clarendon Blvd
Arlington, VA 22209
703 276 8800
www.amerchiro.org

DENTIST (D.D.S., D.M.D.)

Summarized from the *U.S. Bureau of Labor Statistics Occupational Outlook Handbook 2008-2009*. For a complete description, see **www.bls.gov/oco/ocos072.htm**.

I. Career Description

Dentists diagnose and treat diseases of the hard and soft tissue of the mouth. They are also trained to recognize a number of systemic diseases that manifest symptoms within the oral cavity, which would be referred to the appropriate physician. Approximately 80% of the practicing dentists in the U.S. are in a general practice. There are 8 different specialties recognized by the American Dental Association. These are: orthodontics, oral and maxillofacial surgery, endodontics, periodontics, pedodontics, prosthodontics, oral pathology, and dental public health.

II. Career Settings

Most of the 150,000 active dentists in the U.S. today are engaged in private practice. Many have a solo practice, but an increasing number are in group practice. Another trend is for dentists to practice in Health Maintenance Organizations (HMOs) or other corporate entities in which the dentist is an employee rather than the owner of the practice. This is more common among young dentists who are working to accumulate the funds needed to begin their own private practice.

III. Compensation

The average net income for dentists will vary by age and according to whether they are in general practice or a specialty, and whether they are self-employed or employed as an associate by another dentist or a corporate entity. In 2000, the American Dental Education Association reported that the average net income of solo, full-time, private general practitioners was approximately $159,550 per year. For specialists, the average was approximately

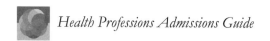
$270,790. Oral surgeons and orthodontists earn well above this average. In 2006, the U.S. Bureau of Labor Statistics reported that the median annual income of salaried dentists was $ 136,960.

IV. Educational Requirements for Practice

Undergraduate Education: 3-4 years, but only about 2% have the minimum 3 years of undergraduate education. The majority will have a baccalaureate degree before entering dental school.

Professional School: 4-year professional degree program that will earn either the D.D.S. or the D.M.D. degree. These two degrees are entirely equivalent in terms of the program taken and the rights conferred for practice.

Graduate Dental Education: Additional postgraduate training is required only for dentists wishing to specialize. General practitioners may enter a practice with no further formal training after the D.M.D. or D.D.S. is conferred.

V. Licensing

All states require dentists to be licensed. In order to obtain a license, the applicant must graduate from an accredited school of dentistry and successfully complete a licensing examination. The Board of Dental Examiners in each state can supply specific information regarding licensure.

VI. Resources

American Dental Association (ADA)
211 East Chicago Avenue
Chicago, IL 60611
312/440-2500
www.ada.org

American Dental Education Association (ADEA)
1400 K Street, NW
Suite 1100
Washington, DC 20005
202/289-7201
www.adea.org

DIETITIANS AND NUTRITIONISTS (R.D)

Summarized from the Bureau of Labor Statistics, U.S. Department of Labor, *Occupational Outlook Handbook, 2008-2009 Edition*, Dietitians and Nutritionists, see **www.bls.gov/oco/ocos077.htm**.

I. Career Description

Dietitians and nutritionists help plan food and nutrition programs, and supervise the preparation and serving of meals. They evaluate the diet of their clients, and suggest modifications to improve health. They may run food service systems for institutions such as schools and hospitals, independently consult with client businesses or individuals, share information through public education programs, and/or conduct related research.

II. Career Settings

In 2006, dieticians and nutritionists held about 57,000 jobs. Many work in hospitals, nursing care facilities and medical clinics. Others are employed in government public health programs, social service agencies, schools, physical fitness facilities, etc.

Employment is expected to grow about as fast as average for all occupations through 2014.

III. Compensation

In 2006, median earnings were $ 46,980, with the middle 50% earning between $ 38,430and $53,370 per year.

IV. Educational Requirements for Practice

Dietitians and nutritionists need at least a bachelor's degree in dietetics, foods and nutrition, food service systems management, or a related area. As of 2007, there were 281 bachelor's degree programs and 22 master's degree programs approved by the American Dietetic Association.

V. Licensing

35 of the 48 States with laws governing dietetics require licensure, 12 require certification and 1 requires registration. Information on licensure is available from state departments of health or boards of occupational licensing.

VI. Resources

American Dietetic Association
120 South Riverside Plaza, Suite 2000
Chicago IL 60606
800/877-1600
www.eatright.org

American Society for Nutrition
9650 Rockville Pike,
Bethesda, MD 20814
301/634-7050
www.asns.org

GENETIC COUNSELOR (M.S.)

Summarized from the National Society of Genetic Counselors (www.nsgc.org) and material from the M.S degree program in Genetic Counseling at the University of North Carolina at Greensboro, see **www.uncg.edu/gen**.

I. Career Description

Genetic counselors are health professionals who have obtained specialized graduate degrees and experience in the areas of medical genetics and counseling. Most have entered the profession from a variety of disciplines, including biology, clinical laboratory science, genetics, nursing, psychology, public health, and social work. Genetic counselors work as members of a health care team to provide information and support to families who have members with birth defects or genetic disorders and to families that may be at risk for a variety of inherited conditions. They identify families at risk, investigate the problem, investigate the problem present in the family, interpret information about the disorder, analyze inheritance patterns and risks of reoccurrence, and review available options with the family. Genetic counselors also provide supportive counseling to families, serve as patient advocates, and refer individuals and families to community or state support agencies. Some counselors work in administrative capacities. Many engage in research related to the fields of medical genetics and genetic counseling.

II. *Career Setting*

Genetic Counselors can work in a variety of setting, which may include some the following: University Medical Centers, Private and Public Hospitals, Diagnostic Laboratories, Physician Private Practices, HMOs, Government Offices, Research and Development/Biotechnology Companies. The primary role of the majority of genetic counselors takes place in a clinical setting.

III. *Compensation*

The average salary for a certified genetic counselor with average work experience was about $60,000 in 2006.

IV. *Educational Requirements for Practice*

The master's degree in Genetic Counseling is the preferred degree in the United States. Programs are also offered in Canada, Australia, England, and South Africa. Courses often include clinical genetics, population genetics, cytogenetics, molecular genetics, psychosocial theory, ethics, and counseling techniques. Programs typically take two years of fulltime study to complete, and include clinical practica in diverse clinical settings.

V. *Licensing*

Certification in Genetic Counseling is available by the American Board of Genetic Counseling (ABGC). Requirements include documentation of the following: a graduate degree in genetic counseling; clinical experience in an ABGC-approved training site or sites; a log book of 50 supervised cases; and successful completion of both the general and specialty certification examination.

VI. *Resources*

National Society of Genetic Counselors
401 N. Michigan Avenue
Chicago, IL 60611
312-321-6834
www.nsgc.org

American Board of Genetic Counseling
P.O. Box 14216
Lenexa, KS 66285
www.abgc.net

HEALTH SERVICES MANAGERS

Summarized from the *U.S. Bureau of Labor Statistics Occupational Outlook Handbook 2008-2009*. For a complete description, see **www.bls.gov/oco/ocos014.htm**.

I. *Career Description*

Health services managers plan, direct, coordinate, and supervise the delivery of health care. Generalists help manage entire facilities or systems, while specialists manage departments or particular services. Increasingly, health services managers are being asked to improve efficiency and reduce costs. Most work long hours.

II. *Career Settings*

Medical and health services managers held about 262,000 jobs in 2006. About 37 percent worked in hospitals, and another 22 percent worked in offices of physicians or in nursing and residential care facilities. Others worked in, home health care agencies, medical clinics, medical laboratories, and a variety of government and private social service agencies.

Employment of health services managers is expected to grow faster than average for all occupations through 2016, as health services continue to expand and diversify.

III. *Compensation*

Median annual earnings of wage and salary medical and health services managers were $73,340 in 2006. The middle 50 percent earned between $57,240 and $94,780. Earnings of medical and health services managers vary widely by type and size of the facility and by level of responsibility

IV. *Educational Requirements for Practice*

A master's degree in health services administration or a related area is the standard credential in this field. A bachelor's degree and/or relevant experience can be adequate for some entry-level positions.

In 2007, 72 schools had accredited programs leading to the master's degree in health services administration, according to the Commission on Accreditation of Healthcare Management Education. There were 42 accredited bachelor's degree programs and 3 master's degree programs in health information management.

V. *Licensing*

All states and the District of Columbia require nursing care facility administrators to have a bachelor's degree, pass a licensing exam, complete a state-approved training program and pursue continuing education. A license is not required in other areas of health services management. Health information managers who have a bachelor's degree or postbaccalaureate from an approved program and who pass an exam can earn certification as a Registered Health Information Administrator from the American Health Information Management Association

VI. *Resources*

American College of Healthcare Executives
One North Franklin Street
Suite 1700
Chicago, IL 60606
312/424-2800
www.ache.org

Association of University Programs in Health Administration
2000 North 14th Street
Suite 780
Arlington, VA 22201
703/894-0940
www.aupha.org

NATUROPATHIC MEDICINE (N.D.)

Summarized from the American Association of Naturopathic Physicians (AANP) website. For a complete description, see: **www.naturopathic.org**

I. *Career Description*

A licensed naturopathic physician is a primary care physician who is trained in the same basic sciences and conventional diagnostics as an M.D., but also specializes in natural, holistic and non-toxic approaches to health care. Emphasis is placed on disease prevention and wellness. The practice of natural therapies includes: Clinical Nutrition, Botanical Medicine, Homeopathic Medicine, Physical Medicine (therapeutic manipulation of muscles and bones), Oriental Medicine, Lifestyle Counseling and Stress Management, and Natural Childbirth, and Minor Surgery.

II. *Career Settings*

Graduates of naturopathic programs work as primary care physicians in private practice and in integrative clinics. Others pursue careers as research scientists, faculty members, natural pharmacists, wellness educators, public health administrators, research and development scientists in the natural products industry, consultants to industry and insurance companies, and advisors to other health care professionals. Naturopathic doctors also function on hospital-based teams with other medical professionals to complement treatments by conventional physicians.

III. *Compensation*

According to a survey conducted by the American Association for Naturopathic Physicians, the income of naturopathic physicians ranges between $55,000 and $200,000. Earnings are comparable to low to mid-range salaries of family practice doctors (approximately $150,000).

IV. *Educational Requirements for Practice*

Academic prerequisites for admission into naturopathic programs include at least three years of pre-medical training and a bachelor's degree. Licensed naturopathic physicians (N.D.) complete a four-year graduate level program at a naturopathic medical school before taking the professional board exam. In addition to the standard medical curriculum in the basic sciences, students are trained in clinical nutrition, acupuncture, homeopathic medicine, botanical medicine, psychology, and counseling. Currently, four U.S. and two Canadian programs are accredited by the Council on Naturopathic Medicine Education (CNME). For a list of accredited and candidate programs, see www.cnme.org/links.html.

V. Licensing

Upon completion of graduate school, a naturopathic physician takes a professional board exam, the Naturopathic Physicians Licensing Exam (NPLEX) so that he or she may be licensed by a state as a primary care general practice physician. Many naturopathic doctors have additional training and certification in acupuncture and home birthing. Currently, thirteen states as well as Puerto Rico and the U.S. Virgin Islands license naturopathic physicians. To view a list of these states, refer to: www.naturopathic.org.

VI. Resources

The American Association of Naturopathic Physicians (AANP)
4435 Wisconsin Avenue, NW
Suite 403
Washington DC 20016
866/538-2267 or 202/ 237-8150
www.naturopathic.org

American Association of Naturopathic Medical Colleges (AANMC)
4435 Wisconsin Avenue, NW
Suite 403
Washington, DC 20016
202/ 237-8150or 866/538-2267
www.aanmc.org/index.php

American Association of Oriental Medicine (AAOM)
PO Box 162340
Sacramento, CA 95816
916/ 443-4770or 866/455-7999
www.aaaomonline.org

Council of Colleges of Acupuncture and Oriental Medicine
3909 National Drive
Suite 125
Burtonsville, MD 20866
301/476-7790
www.ccaom.org

The Naturopathic Medicine Network
www.pandamedicine.com

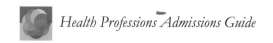

NURSE (B.S.N., M.S.N., Ph.D., D.N.S.)

Summarized from the *U.S. Bureau of Labor Statistics Occupational Outlook Handbook 2084-2009.* For a complete description, see **www.bls.gov/oco/ocos083.htm.**

I. *Career Description*

Registered nurses (R.N.s/B.S.Ns) care for sick people and help them stay well, emotionally as well as physically. The level of a nurse's responsibility depends on the degree held, experience, and advanced education. Nurses may make a nursing diagnosis, which requires observing, assessing, and recording symptoms. They also administer prescribed medications and provide other treatments, usually as directed by the physician. They may work with families, individuals, or groups, in direct nursing roles or as supervisors. Nurses prepared with a master's degree engage in a broad array of advanced practice, clinical specialties, teaching and research. A nurse's duties depend also on the work setting.

Registered nurses constitute the largest health care occupation, with 2.5 million working registered nurses. There is currently a shortage of these health care professionals as "baby boomers" are beginning to retire (*Occupational Outlook Handbook*). Employment of registered nurses is expected to grow much faster than the average for all occupations through 2016.

II. *Career Settings*

Nurses find employment in hospitals, nursing homes, clinics, schools, retirement communities, patients' homes, substance abuse rehabilitation centers, doctors' offices, Health Maintenance Organizations, industry, physical rehabilitation centers, hospices, health departments, governmental agencies, academic institutions, laboratories, administrative offices, and mental health clinics. New niches will develop with time.

III. *Compensation*

According to the *Occupational Outlook Handbook,* median annual earnings of registered nurses were $57,280 in 2006. The middle 50 percent earned between $ 47,710and $ 69,850.

IV. *Educational Requirements for Practice*

There are three options for receiving the necessary credentials after graduation from high school. All require a solid core of biology and chemistry courses:

1. An associate degree (A.D.N. or A.A.) from a community or junior college, usually from a two-year program.

2. A diploma from a hospital school of nursing, usually a two- or three-year program.

3. A baccalaureate degree (B.S.N.) from a college or university, usually a four-year program. The nurse with this degree is the only basic nursing graduate prepared to practice in all health care settings — critical care, ambulatory care, public health, primary care and mental health.

In addition, graduate degrees (M.S.N., Ph.D.) require 2 to 4 years of postbaccalaureate education.

American Association of Colleges of Nursing
One Dupont Circle NW
Suite 530
Washington, DC 20036
202/463-6930
www.aacn.nche.edu

American College of Nurse Practitioners
1501 Wilson Boulevard
Suite 509
 Arlington, VA 22209 703/740-2529
www.acnpweb.org

National League for Nursing (NLN)
61 Broadway, 33rd Floor
New York, NY 10006
800/669-1656
www.nln.org

OCCUPATIONAL THERAPIST (O.T.)

Summarized from the *U.S. Bureau of Labor Statistics Occupational Outlook Handbook 2008-2009*. For a complete description, see **www.bls.gov/oco/ocos078.htm**.

I. *Career Description*

Occupational Therapy involves the social, emotional and physical rehabilitation of people of all ages who are mentally, physically, developmentally, or emotionally challenged. Therapists provide their patients with specialized activities that aid them in mastering the skills necessary to perform daily tasks at home, at work, at school and in the community. The goal is to guide the patient to a life that is as independent, productive and satisfying as possible. Occupational therapy is one of the fastest growing health professions. Those who earn a degree in this area have a high likelihood of finding employment. Current employment opportunities may be lowered by federally mandated limits on reimbursement for therapeutic services; however,), the Bureau of Labor Statistics predicts future growth in the demand for occupational therapists, especially for those working with the elderly.

II. *Career Settings*

The greatest proportion of occupational therapists work in hospitals. Others work in schools and colleges, rehabilitation centers, home health agencies, skilled nursing homes, and private practice. In 2006, there were about 99,000 jobs for OTs according to the *Occupational Outlook Handbook*, published by the Bureau of Labor Statistics (stats.bls.gov/ocohome.htm).

III. *Compensation*

Salaries vary geographically and with the practice setting. In 2006, OTs earned a median salary of about $ 60,470. The middle 50 percent earned between $50,450 and $73,710

IV. Educational Requirements for Practice

A master's degree or higher in occupational therapy is the minimum requirement for entry into the field. In 2007, 124 master's degree programs offered entry-level education, 66 programs offered a combined bachelor's and master's degree, and 5 offered an entry-level doctoral degree Bachelor's degrees in OT are no longer offered. Occupational therapy education may include courses in the physical, biological, and behavioral sciences along with the application of occupational therapy theory and skills. Six months of supervised fieldwork/practicum is required. Relevant undergraduate majors include biology, anthropology, sociology, psychology, and liberal arts. Patience and strong interpersonal skills are necessary for OT practitioners who work in a variety of health care settings.

V. *Licensing*

All States regulate the practice of occupational therapy. For licensing, applicants must graduate from an accredited educational program and pass a national certification examination.

VI. *Resources*

American Occupational Therapy Association, Inc.
4720 Montgomery Lane
P.O. Box 31220
Bethesda, MD 20824-2682
301/652-2682
www.aota.org

OPTOMETRIST (O.D.)

Summarized from the *U.S. Bureau of Labor Statistics Occupational Outlook Handbook 2008-2009*. For a complete description, see **www.bls.gov/oco/ocos073.htm**.

I. *Career Description*

Optometrists are the major providers of primary eye care in the United States. They examine the eyes for vision problems, disease, and other abnormal conditions. They test for proper depth and color perception and the ability to coordinate and focus the eyes, and prescribe lenses and/or treatment. These treatments may include prescription glasses, contact lenses, corrective eye exercises, vision therapy, aids for low vision, and, in some states, therapeutic drugs for specific diseases. They refer patients to the appropriate medical practitioner when related systemic disease is found. Optometrists are also involved in determining preventive vision care for school children, as well as safe vision standards in industry.

II. *Career Settings*

Optometrists work in an office setting. Seventy-one percent of today's practicing optometrists are in an independent practice. A majority of these practice alone, and the rest practice in associate partnerships or group practices. Optometrists may be members of Health Maintenance Organizations; other multidisciplinary group practices, or corporate practices. They also can be found in hospitals and government agencies (e.g. serving as commissioned officers in the Armed Forces), as well as in schools of optometry teaching and doing research. Optometrists held about 33,000 jobs in 2006

III. *Compensation*

The BLS lists median annual earnings of salaried optometrists as $91,040 in 2006. The middle 50 percent earned between $66,530 and $118,490

According to the American Optometric Association, median net annual income for all optometrists, including the self-employed, was $105,000 in 2006. The middle 50 percent earned between $84,000 and $150,000.

IV. *Educational Requirements for Practice*

Undergraduate Education: 3-4 years. Most pre-optometry students enter professional school with a baccalaureate degree.

Professional School: 4-year professional degree program, in a School or College of Optometry.

Graduate Optometric Education: 1-year clinical residency programs are available in some optometric specialties; these include: family practice, pediatric or geriatric optometry, vision training, low vision rehabilitation, contact lenses, and hospital-based and primary care optometry.

V. *Licensing*

All states require that optometrists be licensed. In order to obtain a license, the applicant must have a Doctor of Optometry degree (O.D.) from an accredited School or College of Optometry, and must pass a State Board examination.

Optometrists must renew their licenses annually or biennially, depending upon the state. Most states require some continuing education each year as a requisite for license renewal. The Board of Optometry in each state can supply information regarding licensure.

VI. *Resources*

American Optometric Association (AOA)
243 North Lindbergh Boulevard
St. Louis, MO 63141
800/365-2219
www.aoanet.org

Association of Schools and Colleges of Optometry (ASCO)
6110 Executive Boulevard
Suite 420
Rockville, MD 20852
301/231-5944
www.opted.org

OSTEOPATHIC PHYSICIAN (D.O.)

Summarized from the *U.S. Bureau of Labor Statistics Occupational Outlook Handbook 2008-2009*. For a complete description, see **www.bls.gov/oco/ocos074.htm**.

I. *Career Description*

Osteopathic medicine was developed about 133 years ago as a method of treatment that emphasizes the musculoskeletal system and a concern for the human patient as a complete entity. D.O.s diagnose and treat human diseases and injuries and practice preventive medicine. Some combine medical practice with research or teaching in osteopathic medical schools.

Osteopathic physicians are fully accepted by the public at large and by medical licensing boards in all of the 50 states and the District of Columbia. Residency programs are available to D.O. graduates under the auspices of either the American Osteopathic Association (AOA) or the American Medical Association (AMA). The major distinction between the D.O. and M.D. today is that the D.O. receives specialized training in the treatment method known as Osteopathic Manual Manipulation in addition to the core of medical training common to all physicians, both D.O. and M.D. Secondly, osteopathic medicine emphasizes primary care and a holistic approach to medicine in general. Today, about 65 percent of all osteopathic physicians practice in one of the primary care areas of general practice, pediatrics, obstetrics and gynecology or internal medicine. Even so, osteopathic physicians can be found in virtually all forms of medical practice across the U.S., ranging from general practice in small towns to highly specialized practices in the country's largest cities.

II. *Career Settings*

The D.O. is a licensed physician and may be found in the variety of medical practices commonly known to the general public. While 65% of D.O.s are in primary care areas, many can be found in one of many medical and surgical specialties.

III. *Compensation*

Compensation for the D.O. varies widely, depending on the type of practice, and approximates that of a M.D. in a similar practice, specialty or geographic area. According to the American Association of Colleges of Osteopathic Medicine's (AACOM) 2002 report, the expected starting salary before taxes was approximately $125,000 and rose to about $232,200 after ten years of practice. Incomes are correspondingly higher in specializations and/or large, urban practices.

(Represents median total compensation for allopathic and osteopathic physicians over one year in the specialty in 2005)

Internal Medicine Physicians	$166,420
Surgeons	$282,504
Anesthesiologists	$321,686
Pediatricians	$161,331
Family Practitioners	$156,010
Obstetrics/Gynecology	$247,348

IV. *Educational Requirements for Practice*

Undergraduate Education: All osteopathic medical schools require at least the equivalent of three years of college, but almost all students accepted have a baccalaureate degree and many have advanced degrees. Some osteopathic medical colleges have a combined D.O./Ph.D. degree or a combined D.O./M.S. degree that allows students to obtain both degrees in 4 to 8 years.

Osteopathic Medical Education: 4-year professional degree program in a School of Osteopathic Medicine.

Graduate Osteopathic Education: 12-month rotating internship required of all graduates. The new D.O. may choose to apply for additional work in a variety of residency programs, which may range from 1 to 6 additional years.

V. Licensing

Licensure must be secured in each state. Regardless of the exact method of examination used, licensure in each state in the U.S. carries with it the full range of practice rights and privileges identical with those for M.D. physicians.

VI. Resources

American Association of Colleges of Osteopathic Medicine (AACOM)
5550 Friendship Blvd.
Suite 310
Chevy Chase, MD 20815
301/968-4190
www.aacom.org

American Osteopathic Association (AOA)
142 East Ontario Street
Chicago, IL 60611
800/621-1773
www.osteopathic.org

PHARMACIST (Pharm.D.)

Summarized from the *U.S. Bureau of Labor Statistics Occupational Outlook Handbook 2008-2009*. For a complete description, see **www.bls.gov/oco/ocos079.htm**.

I. Career Description

Pharmacists are health professionals who serve patients and other health professionals in assuring appropriate use of, and optimal therapeutic outcomes from, medications. In addition to the responsibility for professional interpretation and review of prescription orders, medication record screening and review, and the accurate dispensing of medications, pharmacists serve patients and the community by providing information and advice on health, providing medications and associated services, and by referring patients to other sources of help and care, such as physicians, when necessary. According to the Occupational Outlook Handbook, Pharmacists held about 243,000 jobs in 2006. The profession is expected to grow much faster than the average through 2016.

II. Career Settings

Pharmacists typically practice in community pharmacies, chain store pharmacies, hospitals, nursing and long-term care facilities, government agencies and military, educational institutions, and pharmaceutical companies

III. Compensation

Median annual income of wage-and-salary pharmacists in 2006 was $94,520. The middle 50 percent earned between $83,180 and $108,140 a year.

IV. Educational Requirements for Practice

Most students applying to pharmacy school have completed a bachelor's degree. Pharmacists must earn a Pharm.D. degree from an accredited college or school of pharmacy to be eligible for licensure. The Pharm.D. degree has replaced the Bachelor of Pharmacy degree, which is no longer being awarded.

V. Licensing

A license is required in all States, the District of Columbia, and all U.S. territories to receive a license to practice; the pharmacist must have a degree from an accredited pharmacy program and must pass the state's Pharmacy Board Examination.

VI. Resources

American Association of Colleges of Pharmacy (AACP)
1727 King Street
Alexandria, VA 22314
703/739-2330
www.aacp.org

American Society of Health-System Pharmacists (ASHP)
7272 Wisconsin Avenue
Bethesda, MD 20814
301/657-3000
www.ashp.org

American Pharmacists Association (APhA)
1100 15th St. NW
Suite 400
Washington, DC 20005
202/628-4410
www.pharmacist.com

PHYSICIAN ASSISTANT (P.A.)

Summarized from the *U.S. Bureau of Labor Statistics Occupational Outlook Handbook 2008-2009*. For a complete description, see **www.bls.gov/oco/ocos081.htm**.

I. Career Description

The Physician Assistant (PA) is trained in such tasks as screening patients, taking histories, performing physical exams, performing developmental screening exams of children, giving electrocardiograms and blood transfusions, managing emergencies, casting and splinting. A physician willing to accept responsibility may assign more complicated therapeutic procedures to the physician assistant who has demonstrated ability. The PA may also be responsible for keeping records on all patients and for patient follow-up.

Currently the Bureau of Labor Statistics predicts that this is one of the fastest growing careers in the health professions. Physician assistants held about 66,000 jobs in 2006. The BLS expects PA employment to grow much faster than the average for all occupations through the year 2016.

II. Career Settings

Physician Assistants work in physicians' offices, clinics, hospitals, extended care and correctional facilities and Health Maintenance Organizations. Physician Assistants also operate satellite clinics where a physician is present only one day per week and the PA operates the clinic the remaining time.

III. Compensation

The BLS reports median annual earnings of wage-and-salary physician assistants were $74,980 in May 2006. The middle 50 percent earned between $62,430 and $89,220.

According to the American Academy of Physician Assistants, median income for physician assistants in full-time clinical practice was $80,356 in 2006. Income varies by specialty, practice setting, geographical location, and years of experience.

IV. Educational Requirements for Practice

In 2007, 136 education programs for physician assistants were accredited or provisionally accredited by the American Academy of Physician Assistants. More than 90 of these programs offered the option of a master's degree, and the rest offered either a bachelor's degree or an associate degree. Most applicants to PA programs have a bachelor's degree.

While admission requirements vary, most programs require 2 years of college and some hands-on work experience in the health care field. Course work in biology, chemistry, English, mathematics, psychology, and the social sciences is often required for admission. PA schools accept students from diverse experiential backgrounds including nursing, military medics, various allied health professions, and paramedics/EMTs.

V. Licensing

All States and the District of Columbia have legislation governing the qualifications or practice of physician assistants. All jurisdictions require physician assistants to pass the Physician Assistant National Certifying Examination, administered by the National Commission on Certification of Physician Assistants (NCCPA) and open only to graduates of accredited PA education programs.

VI. Resources

Physician Assistant Education Association
300 North Washington Street
Suite 505
Alexandria, VA 22314
703/548-5538
www.paeaonline.org

American Academy of Physician Assistants
950 North Washington Street
Alexandria, VA 22314
703/836-2272
www.aapa.org

PHYSICAL THERAPIST (M.P.T., D.P.T.)

I. Career Description

Physical therapists (PTs) are members of the health care team who provide services that help restore function, improve mobility, relieve pain, and prevent or limit permanent physical disabilities of patients suffering from injuries, disease, and the aging process. They restore, maintain, and promote overall fitness and health. Their patients include accident victims and individuals with disabling conditions such as low-back pain, arthritis, heart disease, fractures, head injuries, and cerebral palsy. The practice of physical therapy involves patient evaluation, treatment and injury prevention. PTs are trained to use a variety of treatment modalities including exercise, manual techniques, the use of ultrasound or electrotherapy, and patient education. There are many areas of specialization within the physical therapy profession.

II. *Career Settings*

Physical therapists work in a variety of settings including hospitals, clinics, private physical therapy offices, home health agencies, skilled nursing facilities, rehabilitation centers, school systems, sports medicine clinics, academic settings (education and research), and government agencies. About two-thirds of physical therapy jobs are either in hospitals or in offices of other health professionals (which includes private PT practices). Physical therapists held about 173,000 jobs in 2006. The number of jobs is greater than the number of practicing physical therapists, because some physical therapists hold two or more jobs. For example, some may work in a private practice, but also work part time in another healthcare facility. The Bureau of Labor Statistics projects much faster than average growth for physical therapy profession through 2016.

III. *Compensation*

Median annual earnings of physical therapists were $66,200 in 2006. The middle 50 percent earned between $55,030 and $78,080. More than 1 in 5 physical therapists worked part time.

IV. *Educational Requirements for Practice*

All states require physical therapists to have graduated from an accredited physical therapist educational program as well as passing a licensure exam. All entry-level PT educational programs minimally award a master's degree with many programs now awarding a Doctor of Physical Therapy (DPT). The vast majority of PT educational programs require applicants to possess a bachelor's degree along with the successful completion of specific prerequisites that can vary from one PT program to another. Common prerequisite requirements may include (but are not limited to): biology, anatomy, physiology, chemistry, physics, statistics, psychology, and other social sciences. As an admission criterion, many PT programs also require some paid or unpaid experience in at least one, if not more, physical therapy settings as well as requiring applicants to take the Graduate Record Exam (GRE). Students seeking entry into a PT program should also have strong interpersonal skills along with a sincere desire to enter a helping profession. Entry into physical therapy programs is competitive. According to the American Physical Therapy Association, there were 209 accredited physical therapist education programs in 2007. Of the accredited programs, 43 offered master's degrees and 166 offered doctoral degrees. Only master's degree and doctoral degree programs are accredited, in accordance with the Commission on Accreditation in Physical Therapy Education. In the future, a doctoral degree might be the required entry-level degree. Master's degree programs typically last 2 years, and doctoral degree programs last 3 years

V. *Resources*

American Physical Therapy Association (APTA)
1111North Fairfax Street
Alexandria, VA 22314-1488
703/684-2782 or 800/999-2782
www.apta.org

PODIATRIC PHYSICIAN (D.P.M.)

Summarized from the *U.S. Bureau of Labor Statistics Occupational Outlook Handbook 2008-2009*. For a complete description, see **www.bls.gov/oco/ocos075.htm**.

I. *Career Description*

The Doctor of Podiatric Medicine is the health professional who deals with the examination, diagnosis, treatment and prevention of diseases and disorders affecting the feet and lower leg. Doctors of Podiatric Medicine share with other physicians the legal authority to make independent professional judgments and to administer medical and surgical treatment.

Podiatrists held about 12,000 jobs in 2006. About 24 percent of podiatrists were self-employed. Most podiatrists were solo practitioners, although more are entering partnerships and multispecialty group practices.

II. *Career Settings*

The demand for podiatric medical services is growing rapidly. Modern emphasis on physical fitness and recreational activities such as jogging, running and hiking are placing greater demands on our feet and their appropriate care. Podiatrists are licensed to practice in all fifty states, the District of Columbia and Puerto Rico. Podiatrists serve on the staffs of hospitals, as faculty in health professions schools, in public health programs, as commissioned officers in the Armed Forces and in private practice.

III. *Compensation*

The BLS reports median annual earnings of salaried podiatrists were $108,220 in 2006. A survey by *Podiatry Management Magazine* reported median net income of $114,000 in 2006.

IV. *Educational Requirements for Practice*

Undergraduate Education: All colleges of podiatric medicine require a minimum of three years (90 semester hours) of premedical education; 95% of students matriculating into schools of Podiatry have a baccalaureate degree.

Professional School: 4-year professional degree program in a School or College of Podiatric Medicine.

Graduate Medical Education: 1 to 2 years of residency training.

V. *Licensing*

A Doctor of Podiatric Medicine (D.P.M.) is required for practice. Licensure is granted upon successfully passing an examination by the state and/or National Board of Podiatry Examiners.

VI. *Resources*

American Association of Colleges of Podiatric Medicine (AACPM)
15850 Crabbs Branch Way
Suite 320
Rockville, MD 20855
800/922-9266
www.aacpm.org

American Podiatric Medical Association (APMA)
9312 Old Georgetown Road
Bethesda, MD 20814
301/581-9200
www.apma.org

PUBLIC HEALTH (M.P.H., Ph. D.)

Summarized from the *U.S. Bureau of Labor Statistics Occupational Outlook Handbook 2008-2009*. For a complete description, see **www.bls.gov/oco**.

I. *Career Description*

Rather than focussing on individuals, public health care workers endeavor to protect and improve the health of whole groups of people. They assess and monitor the health of populations, educate decision makers and the public, and develop and implement policies and programs. Public health is a multi-disciplinary field involving many different kinds of professionals, including some physicians and nurses, as well as graduates of formal public health programs. There is also a wide variety of specialty areas within the field, including biostatistics, epidemiology, environmental health, health education, health services administration, international public health, nutrition and occupational health and safety.

II. *Career Settings*

Depending on their specialty, public health workers may be employed by government agencies and health departments, insurance companies, community wellness centers, public school systems, colleges and universities, hospitals, private businesses or other facilities.

III. *Compensation*

ASPH notes that because public health professionals work in such a wide variety of settings and are often work in multi-disciplinary capacities, the salaries vary significantly from job to job. There is currently no national data available to ASPH on the average starting salary that is representative of what a graduate can expect. ASPH refers potential MPH students to www.publichealthjobs.net for information on particular positions

According to the Association of Schools of Public Health, in 2002 recent starting salaries within one year of graduation from a public health program were $37,050–$161,400 for health services administrators, $33,000–$63,000 for bio-statisticians, $38,175–$136,237 for epidemiology specialists, $33,000–$86,625 for health educators/behavioral scientists, $44,550–$143,700 for environmental health scientists, and $31,500–$86,625 for international public health specialists. There is currently demand for public health workers in epidemiology, biostatistics, some environmental and occupational health specialties, public health nutrition, public health nursing, and public health and preventive medicine. (Source: www.asph.org/document.cfm?page=727#average%20salary)

IV. *Educational Requirements for Practice*

A master's degree in public health (M.P.H.) or related area is a typical credential in this field, though educational requirements vary depending on the profession and specialty area.

V. Licensing

Licensure and certification requirements vary, depending on the specialty area.

VI. Resources

Association of Schools of Public Health
1101 15th Street NW
Suite 910
Washington, DC 20005
202/296-1099
www.asph.org

American Public Health Association
800 I Street NW
Washington, DC 20001
202/777-2742
www.apha.org

RECREATIONAL THERAPIST

Summarized from the *U.S. Bureau of Labor Statistics Occupational Outlook Handbook 2004-2005*. For a complete description, see **www.bls.gov/oco/ocos082.htm**.

I. Career Description

Recreational therapists, also referred to as therapeutic recreation specialists, provide treatment services and recreation activities to people with disabilities or illnesses. They assess client needs and interests, and develop and carry out interventions. Treatments may include the use of arts and crafts, animals, sports, games, dance and movement, drama, music and/or community outings.

II. Career Settings

Recreational therapists held about 25,000 jobs in 2006. About 70 percent were in nursing and residential care facilities and hospitals. Others worked in settings such as community mental health centers, correctional facilities and adult day care programs.

The BLS predicts that employment of recreational therapists will grow more slowly than the average for all occupations through the year 2016.

III. Compensation

Median annual earnings of recreational therapists were $34,990 in 2006. The middle 50 percent earned between $26,780 and $44,850. Those employed in hospitals had the highest incomes.

IV. Educational Requirements for Practice

A bachelor's degree in therapeutic recreation, or in recreation with a concentration in therapeutic recreation, is the usual requirement for entry-level positions. There are approximately 150 associate, bachelors, masters and doctoral degree programs.

V. Licensing

Most employers prefer to hire candidates who are certified therapeutic recreation specialists (CTRS).

VI. Resources

American Therapeutic Recreation Association
207 3rd Avenue
Hattiesburg, MS 39401
601-450-2872
atra-online.com/cms

National Therapeutic Recreation Society (now a branch of the National Recreation and Park Association)
22377 Belmont Ridge Road
Ashburn, VA 20148
703/858-0784 or 800/626-6772
www.nrpa.org

RESPIRATORY THERAPIST

Summarized from the *U.S. Bureau of Labor Statistics, Occupational Outlook Handbook, 2008-2009*. For a complete description, see **www.bls.gov/oco/ocos084.htm**.

I. Career Description

Respiratory therapists (also known as respiratory care practitioners) specialize in the treatment of individuals with breathing or other cardiopulmonary disorders. They work closely with physicians and other health care professionals to develop and modify individual patient care plans. Treatments include: oxygen therapy, chest physiotherapy, and aerosol medications.

II. Career Settings

Respiratory therapists work primarily in hospitals. Their traditional roles are expanding into areas such as pulmonary rehabilitation, smoking cessation counseling, disease prevention, and even sleep disorders. They play an important role in critical care medicine.

The BLS predicts faster than average growth through 201 for respiratory therapists. The increasing demand will come from substantial growth in the middle-aged and elderly population — a development that will heighten the incidence of cardiopulmonary disease

III. Compensation

Median annual earnings of wage-and-salary respiratory therapists were $47,420 in May 2006. The middle 50 percent earned between $40,840 and $56,160.

IV. Educational Requirements for Practice

An associate degree is the minimum educational requirement, but a bachelor's or master's degree may be important for advancement. Training is offered at the college/university level, medical schools, vocational/technical institutes, and the Armed Forces. According to the Commission on Accreditation of Allied Health Education Programs (CAAHEP), 45 entry-level and 334 advanced respiratory therapy programs were accredited in the United States in 2006.

V. Licensing

A license is required to practice as a respiratory therapist, except in Alaska and Hawaii. Also, most employers require respiratory therapists to maintain a cardiopulmonary resuscitation (CPR) certification. Licensure is usually based, in large part, on meeting the requirements for certification from the National Board for Respiratory Care (NBRC).

VI. Resources

American Association for Respiratory Care
9425 N. MacArthur Blvd.
Suite 100
Irving, TX 75063
972/243-2272
www.aarc.org

Commission on Accreditation for Allied Health Education Programs
1361 Park St.
Clearwater, FL 33756
727/210-2350
www.caahep.org

SPEECH-LANGUAGE PATHOLOGIST AND AUDIOLOGIST

Summarized from the *U.S. Bureau of Labor Statistics, Occupational Outlook Handbook 2008-2009*. For a complete description, see **www.bls.gov/oco/ocos099.htm**.

I. Career Description

Speech-language pathologists assess, treat, and help to prevent speech, language, cognitive, communication, voice, swallowing, fluency, and other disorders. They work with people who cannot clearly make speech sounds; those with rhythm or fluency problems, such as stuttering; those with voice quality problems, such as inappropriate pitch or harshness; those with problems understanding language; and those with cognitive communication impairments.

Audiologists identify, assess, and manage auditory, balance, and other neural systems. They work with people who have hearing, balance and related problems.

II. Career Settings

Speech-language pathologists held about 110,000 jobs in 2006. About one-half worked in schools or colleges. Others worked in hospitals, medical practices, hearing centers, home health agencies or other facilities. Audiologists held about 12,000 jobs in 2006. More than half of all jobs were in health care facilities.

The BLS expects employment for both professions to grow about as fast as the average for all occupations through 2016.

III. Compensation

Median annual earnings of wage-and-salary speech-language pathologists were $57,710 in May 2006. The middle 50 percent earned between $46,360 and $72,410. Those in health care settings earned substantially more than those practicing in schools. Median annual earnings of wage-and-salary audiologists were $57,120 in May 2006. The middle 50 percent earned between $47,220 and $70,940.

IV. Educational Requirements for Practice

Most speech-language pathologist jobs require a master's degree. In 2007, more than 230 colleges and universities offered graduate programs in speech-language pathology accredited by the Council on Academic Accreditation in Audiology and Speech-Language Pathology. Most states require a master's degree or equivalent for licensure. About 239 colleges and universities offer graduate programs in speech pathology, and about 86 offer graduate audiology programs. All States require audiologists to be licensed or registered. Licensure or registration requires at least a master's degree in audiology; however, a first professional, or doctoral, degree is becoming increasingly necessary.

V. Licensing

In 2007, 47 States regulated speech-language pathologists through licensure or registration. Requirements may vary depending on the setting in which the pathologist will practice. , Audiologists are regulated by licensure or registration in all 50 States.audiologists.   Information on licensure is available from state departments of health or boards of occupational licensing.

VI. Resources

American Speech-Language-Hearing Association
2200 Research Boulevard
Rockville, MD 20850
301-296-5700
www.asha.org

American Academy of Audiology
11730 Plaza America Drive
Suite 300
Reston, VA 20190
800/AAA-2336
www.audiology.org

VETERINARIAN (D.V.M.)

Summarized from the *U.S. Bureau of Labor Statistics Occupational Outlook Handbook 2008-2009*. For a complete description, see **www.bls.gov/oco/ocos076.htm**.

I. Career Description

Veterinarians diagnose, treat, and control diseases in animals and are concerned with preventing the transmission of animal diseases to humans. Also, they treat injured animals and develop programs to prevent disease and injury. Veterinarians held about 62,000 jobs in 2006.

II. Career Settings

According to the American Veterinary Medical Association, about 3 out of 4 veterinarians were employed in a solo or group practice Veterinarians in private practice may limit the species of animals they normally treat to dogs, cats, birds, other domesticated pets, horses, farm animals, or exotics. Others serve with wildlife management groups, zoos, aquariums, and animal shelters. All may supervise Veterinary Assistants and Technicians. Many are employed by city, country, state or federal government agencies that investigate, test for and control diseases in livestock and poultry, which affect both animal and human health. Pharmaceutical and biomedical research firms seek veterinarians to develop, test and supervise the production of drugs, chemicals and biological products such as serums and vaccines that are designed for human and animal use. Still other veterinarians are engaged in research and teaching at veterinary and medical schools, working for racetracks or other animal-related enterprises and within the military. The profession is expected to grow much faster than average through 2016.

III. Compensation

Veterinarians' salaries are based on length of time since graduation, location, and level and type of specialization. According to BLS, Median annual earnings of veterinarians were $71,990 in 2006. The middle 50 percent earned between $56,450 and $94,880. The average annual salary for veterinarians in the Federal Government was $84,335 in 2007.

IV. Educational Requirements for Practice

Undergraduate Education: Most veterinary schools require at least the equivalent of 3 years of college; some require a baccalaureate degree. Most students enter with at least a bachelor's degree, and some have advanced degrees.

Professional School: 4-year professional degree program.

Graduate Veterinary Medical Education: 1 to 4 years of residency training. Veterinarians who wish to teach or conduct research may earn a Ph.D. degree.

V. Licensing

State Board examinations are given by the state in which a veterinarian wishes to practice. The American Veterinary Medical Association recognizes specialties in the following areas: anesthesiology, cardiology, dermatology, epidemiology, equine, internal medicine (neurology, ophthalmology), laboratory animal medicine, microbiology, pathology, preventive medicine, radiology, surgery, theriogenology, toxicology, veterinary practice (companion animals, food animals), and zoological medicine. Other specialties are currently under review for board certification. Internships and residency programs of varying lengths of time provide the training for these specialties, after which the board examinations are taken and certification is granted.

VI. Resources

American Veterinary Medical Association (AVMA)
1931 North Meacham Road
Suite 100
Schaumburg, IL 60173
847/925-8070
avma.org

Association of American Veterinary Medical Colleges (AAVMC)
1101 Vermont Avenue NW
Suite 301
Washington, DC 20005
202/371-9195
www.aavmc.org

Veterinary Information Network
777 West Covell Blvd
Davis, CA 95616
800/700-4636 or 530/756-4881
www.vin.com

The Bureau of Labor Statistics lists a full category of health careers that does not require a bachelor's degree as those listed above do. These careers are listed below. Visit the BLS website and Health technnologists and technicians for specific information about them. For a complete description, see www.bls.gov/oco/oco1002.htm.

Athletic trainers
Cardiovascular technologists and technicians
Clinical laboratory technologists and technicians
Dental hygienists
Diagnostic medical sonographers
Emergency medical technicians and paramedics
Licensed practical and licensed vocational nurses
Medical records and health information technicians
Nuclear medicine technologists
Occupational health and safety specialists and technicians
Opticians, dispensing
Pharmacy technicians
Radiologic technologists and technicians
Surgical technologists
Veterinary technologists and technicians

Appendix B

Health Professions Acronyms, and Organizations

ALPHABETICAL LISTING OF ACRONYMS

AACN	American Association of Colleges of Nursing
AACOM	American Association of Colleges of Osteopathic Medicine
AACOMAS	American Association of Colleges of Osteopathic Medicine Application Service
AACP	American Association of Colleges of Pharmacy
AACPM	American Association of Colleges of Podiatric Medicine
AADSAS	American Association of Dental Schools Application Service
AANP	American Association of Naturopathic Medicine
AANP	American Association of Naturopathic Medicine
AAMC	Association of American Medical Colleges
AAVMC	Association of American Veterinary Medical Colleges
ACA	American Chiropractic Association
ACOE	Accreditation Council on Optometric Education
ACT	American College Testing Program
ADA	American Dental Association
ADEA	American Dental Education Association
AED	Alpha Epsilon Delta
ASDA	American Student Dental Association
AHA	American Hospital Association
AHPAT	Allied Health Professions Admission Test
ALP	Alternative Loan Program
AMA	American Medical Association
AMCAS	American Medical College Application Service
AMSA	American Medical Student Association
ANA	American Nurses Association
AOA	American Optometric Association
AOA	American Osteopathic Association
AOTA	American Occupational Therapy Association
APhA	American Pharmacists Association
APTA	American Physical Therapy Association
APMA	American Podiatric Medicine Association
APHA	American Public Health Association
ASCO	Association of Schools and Colleges of Optometry
ASPH	Association of Schools of Public Health
AVMA	American Veterinary Medical Association
CDC	Centers for Disease Control, Public Health Service, Health and Human Services
COA	Committee on Admissions — GSA, AAMC
COD	Council of Deans — AAMC

CAAHEP	Commission on Accreditation of Allied Health Education Programs
COSA	Committee on Student Affairs — GSA, AAMC
COSFA	Committee on Student Financial Assistance — GSA, AAMC
COGME	Council on Graduate Medical Education
COTH	Council of Teaching Hospitals — AAMC
DAT	Dental Admission Test
DEAL	Dental Education Assistance Loan
DRG	Diagnostic Related Group
ECFMG	Educational Commission for Foreign Medical Graduates
EFN	Exceptional Financial Need (scholarship program)
ETS	Educational Testing Service
FADHPS	Financial Assistance to Disadvantaged Health Professions Students (scholarship program)
FLEX	Federal Licensing Examination
FMG	Foreign Medical Graduate
FMGEMS	Foreign Medical Graduate Examination in the Medical Sciences
GAPSFAS	Graduate and Professional School Financial Aid Service — ETS
GEA	Group of Educational Affairs — AAMC
GME	Group on Medical Education — AAMC, section of GEA
GRE	Graduate Record Exam
GSA	Group on Student Affairs — AAMC
GSL	Guaranteed Student Loan (now known as the Stafford Loan)
HHS	Health and Human Services (Department of)
HMO	Health Maintenance Organization
HPSL	Health Professions Student Loans
HPSP	Health Professions Scholarship Program (Army, Navy, Air Force)
IAB	International Association of Boards of Examiners in Optometry
ICL	Income Contingent Loan
LCME	Liaison Committee on Medical Education
MAS	Minority Affairs Section — AAMC, section of GSA
MCAT	Medical College Admission Test
MSOP	Medical School Objectives Project — AAMC
MSTP	Medical Scientist Training Program
NAAHP	National Association of Advisors for the Health Professions
NACADA	National Academic Advising Association
NAMME	National Association of Medical Minority Educators
NBEO	National Board of Examiners in Optometry
NBME	National Board of Medical Examiners
NCI	National Cancer Institute — NIH
NDSL	National Direct Student Loan (now known as the Perkins Loan)
NHLBI	National Heart, Lung and Blood Institute — NIH
NHSC	National Health Service Corps — HHS
NIGMS	National Institute of General Medical Sciences — NIH
NIH	National Institutes of Health
NLM	National Library of Medicine — NIH
NLN	National League for Nursing
NMA	National Medical Association
NMF	National Medical Fellowships
NRMP	National Residency Matching Program
OAT	Optometry Admission Test

OSR	Organization of Student Representatives — AAMC
PAEA	Physician Assistant Education Association
PCAT	Pharmacy College Admission Test
PHARMCAS	Pharmacy College Application Service
PHS	Public Health Service
PPO	Preferred Provider Organization
PRO	Peer Review Organization
SLS	Supplemental Loan to Students
SMDEP	Summer Medical & Dental Education Program
SNMA	Student National Medical Association
USMLE	United States Medical Licensing Examination (I, II, and III Steps)
VMCAS	Veterinary Medical College Application Service
VQE	Visa Qualifying Exam
WWAMI	Washington, Wyoming, Alaska, Montana, Idaho Medical Education Program
WICHE	Western Interstate Commission on Higher Education

ORGANIZATIONS GROUPED BY FUNCTION

Professional Organizations

ACA	American Chiropractic Association
ADA	American Dental Association
AHA	American Hospital Association
AMA	American Medical Association
AMSA	American Medical Student Association
ANA	American Nurses Association
APhA	American Pharmacists Association
AOA	American Optometric Association
AOA	American Osteopathic Association
APA	American Podiatry Association
AVMA	American Veterinary Medical Association
NLN	National League for Nursing
NMA	National Medical Association
SNMA	Student National Medical Association
AOSA	American Optometric Student Association

Professional School Associations

AACOM	American Association of Colleges of Osteopathic Medicine
AACP	American Association of Colleges of Pharmacy
AACPM	American Association of Colleges of Podiatric Medicine
AANP	American Association of Naturopathic Medicine
AAMC	Association of American Medical Colleges
AAVMC	Association of American Veterinary Medical Colleges
ADEA	American Dental Education Association
APTA	American Physical Therapy Association
ASCO	Association of Schools and Colleges of Optometry
ASPH	Association of Schools of Public Health
PAEA	Physician Assistant Education Association

Tests

DAT	Dental Admission Test
ECFMG	Educational Commission for Foreign Medical Graduates
FMGEMS	Foreign Medical Graduate Examination in the Medical Sciences
GRE	Graduate Record Exam
MCAT	Medical College Admission Test
OAT	Optometry Admission Test
PCAT	Pharmacy College Admission Test
TOEFL	Test of English as Foreign Language
USMLE	United States Medical Licensing Exam (I, II, and III Steps)

Testing and Certification Groups/Sponsors

ACT	American College Testing Program
ETS	Educational Testing Service
ECFMG	Educational Commission for Foreign Medical Graduates
FLEX	Federal Licensing Examination (Once lead to licensure in medicine)
GAPSFAS	Graduate and Professional School Financial Aid Service (sponsored by ETS; does need analysis for scholarships and loans)

Government Organizations with Health Care/Research/Regulatory Responsibilities

CDC	Center for Disease Control and Prevention, Department of Health and Human Services
NIH	National Institutes of Health composed of several different institutes, including:
NIAID	National Institute of Allergy and Infectious Diseases
NCI	National Cancer Institute
NIMH	National Institutes of Mental Health
NIDR	National Institute of Dental Research
NLM	National Library of Medicine
NHSC	National Health Service Corps
PHS	Public Health Service

Loan and Scholarship Programs

ALP	Alternative Loan Program (AAMC)
DEAL	Dental Education Assistance Loan
EFN	Exceptional Financial Need (scholarship)
FADHPS	Financial Assistance to Disadvantaged Health Professions Students (scholarship)
GSL	Guaranteed Student Loan (Stafford Loan)
HPSL	Health Professions Student Loan
HPSP	Health Professions Scholarship Program (military scholarship awarded by Army, Navy and Air Force)
MEDLOANS	An umbrella loan coordinating program sponsored by AAMC
MSTP	Medical Scientist Training Program (NIH-sponsored grant for students in M.D./Ph.D. joint degree programs)
NDSL	National Direct Student Loan, now called Perkins Loan
NMF	National Medical Fellowships, Inc., an organization that provides scholarships to minority students

AAMC-Sponsored Organizations and Activities

ALP	Alternative Loan Program
AMCAS	American Medical College Application Service
COA, GSA	Committee on Admissions, Group on Student Affairs
COD	Council of Deans
COSA-GSA	Committee on Student Affairs, Group on Student Affairs
COTH	Council of Teaching Hospitals
GME	Group on Medical Education
GSA	Group on Student Affairs
MAS	Minority Affairs Section
MEDLOANS	An umbrella loan program
OSR	Organization of Student Representatives
MSAR	A book published yearly listing requirements for all LCME-accredited medical schools (see LCME listed below)

Medical Groups Other than School or Professional

DRG	Diagnostic Related Group, a method used to determine payment for medical treatment/hospital stays
HMO	Health Maintenance Organization, a company organized to provide prepaid medical care for a group
PPO	Preferred Provider Organization, a group practice that will give fee discounts to patients who are employees of a contracting company, union, etc
PRO	Peer Review Organization, a group composed primarily of physicians who work under government contract to monitor hospital care of Medicare patients.
RBRVS	Resource Based Relative Value Scale, a new system for determining payment to physicians under Medicare

Other Groups Not Listed Above

LCME	Liaison Committee on Medical Education is the accrediting organization for medical schools, made up of representatives from the AMA and AAMC.
GMENAC	The Graduate Medical Education National Advisory Committee in 1981 published a controversial report predicting a large surplus of physicians by 1995.
GPEP	The Graduate and Professional Education of the Physician and College Preparation for Medicine study was made over a three-year period by a 19-person committee. Whether the published recommendations have had any appreciable impact on medical education is debatable.
MSOP	The Medical School Objectives Project provided a self-assessment of medical education that resulted in objectives to guide medical schools in reevaluating and reforming their curricula.
NRMP	The National Residency Matching Program conducts "The Match" each March, by assigning fourth-year medical students to their residency positions for the coming year.
WICHE	The Western Interstate Commission for Higher Education administers contract positions in the West, especially for states such as Idaho, Montana, Alaska, etc. that do not have medical schools.

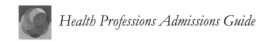

PRACTITIONER ASSOCIATIONS

Listed below are some of the general practitioner associations:
American Academy of Physician Assistants
American College of Health Care Administrators
American Dental Association
American Medical Association
American Optometric Association
American Osteopathic Association
American Pharmacists Association
American Physical Therapy Association
American Podiatric Medical Association
American Public Health Association
American Veterinary Medical Association

Application Services

American Association of Colleges of Osteopathic Medicine Application Service:

AACOMAS
5550 Friendship Boulevard, Suite 310
Chevy Chase, MD 20815

Phone: 301/968-4190
Email: aacomas@aacom.org
Web: www.aacom.org

American Association of Colleges of Podiatric Medicine Application Service:

AACPMAS
15850 Crabbs Branch Way, Suite 320
Rockville, MD 20855

Phone: 800/922-9266
Email: aacpmas@aacpm.org
Web: www.e-aacpmas.org

American Association of Dental Schools Application Service:

AADSAS
1400 K Street NW, Suite 1100
Washington, DC 20005-2212

Phone: 202/289-8123
800/353-2237
Applicants only: 617/612-2045
Web: www.adea.org

American Medical College Application Service:

AMCAS
2450 N Street, NW
Washington, DC 20037

Phone: 202/828-0600
Email: amcas@aamc.org
Web: www.aamc.org

Central Application Service for Physician Assistants:

CASPA
PO Box 9108
Watertown, MA 02471
Web: caspaonline.org

Phone: 617/612-2080
Email: caspainfo@caspaonline.org

Optometry Centralized Application Service:

OptomCAS – To Launch July 15, 2009
6110 Executive Boulevard, Suite 420
Rockville, MD 20852

Phone: 301/231-5944 ext 3019
Fax: 301/770-1824
Email: ppence@opted.org
Web: www.optomcas.org

Pharmacy College Application Service:

PharmCAS
PO Box 9108
Watertown, MA 02472

Phone: 703/739-2330
Fax: 703/836-8982
Email: info@pharmcas.org
Web: www.pharmcas.org

Physical Therapist Centralized Application Service:

PTCAS
PO Box 9112
Watertown, MA 02471

Phone: 617/612-2040
Email: ptcasinfo@ptcas.org
Web: www.ptcas.org

Schools of Public Health Application Service:

SOPHAS
PO Box 9111
Watertown, MA 02471

Phone: 617/612-2090
Email: sophasinfo@sophas.org
Web: www.sophas.org

Veterinary Medical College Application Service:

VMCAS
1101 Vermont Avenue, NW, Suite 301
Washington, DC 20005

Phone: 202/682-0750
Student/Advisor Hotline: 877/862-2740
Email: vmcas@aavmc.org
Web: www.aavmc.org

Admission Test Dates for Graduate & Professional Schools

Test	Test Date	Application Registration Deadline (Standard U.S.)
Dental Admissions Test (DAT) Dental Admissions Testing Program American Dental Association 211 East Chicago Avenue, 6th Floor Chicago, IL 60611 800/232-2162 email: education@ada.org www.ada.org	Computerized tests are available almost every business day.	Applicants must register in advance of test date.
Graduate Record Exam (GRE) Educational Testing Service PO Box 6000 Princeton, NJ 08541-6000 866/473-4373 www.gre.org	Computerized tests are available year round	Applicants must register in advance by calling:1-800-GRE-CALL
Medical College Admission Test (MCAT) MCAT Program Office PO Box 4056 Iowa City, IA 52243 319/337-1357 email: mcat_reg@act.org www.aamc.org/mcat	Computerized tests are offered at various times throughout the year.	Applicants must register in advance of test date.
Optometry Admission Test (OAT) Optometry Admission Testing Program 211 East Chicago Avenue, 6th Floor Chicago, IL 60611-2678 800/232-2159 www.opted.org	Computerized tests are available almost every business day.	Applicants must register in advance of test date.
Pharmacy College Admission Test (PCAT) Pearson Customer Relations - PCAT 19500 Bulverde Road San Antonio, TX 78259 800/622-3231; fax: 888/211-8276 www.pcatweb.info	June 20, 2009 August 22, 2009 October 17, 2009 January 23, 2010	May 8, 2009 July 10, 2009 September 4, 2009 December 11, 2009

ORGANIZATIONS OF ADVISORS FOR THE HEALTH PROFESSIONS

National Association

National Association of Advisors for the Health Professions, Inc. (NAAHP)
P.O. Box 1518
Champaign, IL   61824-1518
217/355-0063
www.naahp.org
NAAHPja@aol.com

Regional Associations

Central Association of Advisors for the Health Professions (CAAHP)   www.caahp.org
Northeast Association of Advisors for the Health Professions (NEAAHP)   www.neaahp.org
Southeastern Association of Advisors for the Health Professions (SAAHP)   www.saahp.org
Western Association of Advisors for the Health Professions (WAAHP)   www.waahp.org

SELECTED ORGANIZATIONS FOR STUDENTS

Alpha Epsilon Delta — the Premedical Honor Society
James Madison University
601 University Boulevard
MSC 9015
Harrisonburg, VA 22807
540/568-2594
www.nationalaed.org

American Student Dental Association
Suite 700
211 East Chicago Avenue
Chicago, IL 66061
800/621-8099, ext. 2795
www.asdanet.org

American Medical Student Association (open to premedical students)
1902 Association Drive
Reston, VA 20191
703/620-6600
www.amsa.org

Academy of Students of Pharmacy
American Pharmacists Associationp
1100 15th Street NW
Suite 400
Washington, DC 20005
202/628-4410
www.pharmacist.com

Student National Medical Association (open to premedical students)
5113 Georgia Ave. NW
Washington, DC 20011
202/882-2881
www.snma.org

SCHOOL AND PRACTITIONER ORGANIZATIONS

Career	*Health Professional School Association*	*Practitioner Association*
Allopathic Medicine	Association of American Medical Colleges 2450 N Street NW Washington, DC 20037	American Medical Association 515 North State Street Chicago, IL 60610
Chiropractic	Association of Chiropractic Colleges 4424 Montgomery Ave. Suite 102 Bethesda, MD 20814	
Dentistry	American Dental Education Association 1400 K Street NW, Suite 1100 Washington, DC 20005	American Dental Association 211 East Chicago Avenue Chicago, IL 60611-2678
Naturopathic Medicine	American Association of Naturopathic Medical Colleges 4435 Wisconsin Ave NW, Suite 403 Washington, DC 20016	American Assoc of Naturopathic Physicians 4435 Wisconsin Ave NW, Suite 403 Washington, DC 20016
Nursing	American Association of Colleges of Nursing One Dupont Circle NW, Suite 530 Washington, DC 20036	National League For Nursing 61 Broadway, 33rd floor New York, NY 10006
Optometry	Assoc. of Schools & Colleges of Optometry 6110 Executive Boulevard, Suite 420 Rockville, MD 20852	American Optometric Association 243 North Lindbergh Boulevard St. Louis , MO 63141
Osteopathic Medicine	Amer. Assoc. of Colleges of Osteopathic Med. 5550 Friendship Blvd. , Suite 310 Chevy Chase, MD 20815-7231	American Osteopathic Association 142 East Ontario Street Chicago, IL 60611
Pharmacy	American Association of Colleges of Pharmacy 1426 Prince Street Alexandria, VA 22314	American Pharmacists Association 1727 King St. 1100 15th Street NW, Suite 400 Washington, DC 20005
Physical Therapy		American Physical Therapy Association 1111 North Fairfax Street Alexandria, VA 22314-1488

Physician Assistant	Physician Assistant Education Association 950 North Washington Street, Suite 505 Alexandria, VA 22314 -2544	American Academy of Physician Assistants 950 North Washington Street Alexandria, VA 22314-1552
Podiatric Medicine	Amer. Assoc. of Colleges of Podiatric Medicine 15850 Crabbs Branch Way, Suite 320 Rockville, MD 20855	American Podiatric Medical Association 9312 Old Georgetown Road Bethesda, MD 20814-1621
Public Health	Association of Schools of Public Health 1101 15th Street NW, Suite 910 Washington, DC 20005	American Public Health Association 800 I Street NW Washington, DC 20001-3710
Veterinary Medicine	Assoc. of American Veterinary Medical Colleges 1101 Vermont Avenue NW, Suite 301 Washington, DC 20005	American Veterinary Medical Association 1931 North Meacham Road, Suite 100 Schaumburg

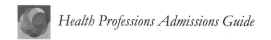

APPENDIX C
REFERENCE MATERIALS

- *300 Ways to Put Your Talent to Work in the Health Field.* A booklet that gives information about virtually every health career. National Health Council. www.nationalhealthcouncil.org

- *AACPM Colleges of Podiatric Medicine College Information Booklet.* American Association of Colleges of Podiatric Medicine. www.aacpm.org or call 800/922-9266.

- *ADEA Official Guide to Dental Schools* (revised annually in late winter). Lists each school by state, giving admission requirements, selection factors, etc. American Dental Education Association (ADEA). www.adea.org

- *Health Professions Career and Education Directory,* 2007-2008. Contains information on nearly 6,900 allied health educational programs and 2,500 sponsoring institutions in the U.S. Published by the American Medical Association (AMA). www.ama-assn.org

- *Keepsake: A Guide for Minority PreMed Students.* Guide for minority students interested in the health professions. Spectrum Unlimited. www.minoritymedicalstudents.com

- *Medical School Admission Requirements* (U.S. and Canada; revised annually in April). Lists each AAMC school by state, giving admission requirements, selections factors, acceptance data and the name of the admissions officer. Association of American Medical Colleges. www.aamc.org

- *MD²: Monetary Decisions for Medical Doctors* , *Financial Education and Wellness (FEW)*, and *Medloans.* Information on financial planning for medical school and on loans available to help finance medical education. AAMC. www.aamc.org (free).

- *Minority Student Opportunities in U.S. Medical Schools* (revised biennially). Includes information on recruitment programs, admission policies, academic assistance programs and financial aid programs for minority students. AAMC. www.aamc.org

- *Nursing Programs 2009.* 14th edition, Peterson's, 2006. www.petersons.com; sold through amazon.com

- *Opportunities for Minority Students: United States Dental Schools 2006-08.* Washington D.C.: Association of American Dental Schools. www.adea.org

- *Physician Assistant Programs Directory.* Purchase access to this online resource at www.paeaonline.org

- *Schools and Colleges of Optometry: Admission Requirements.* Profiles of each school of optometry are included. The booklet also provides general information about the profession and guidelines for a course of study. American Optometric Association . www.opted.org

- *Osteopathic Medical College Information Book.*(revised annually) Available from American Association of Colleges of Osteopathic Medicine (AACOM) in print or online. Contains current information about member colleges of AACOM. Lists colleges of osteopathic medicine; also lists other publications from AACOM. www.aacom.org

- *Pharmacy School Admission Requirements,*. (revised annually). Lists U.S. pharmacy schools by state; includes admission requirements and other helpful information. American Association of Colleges of Pharmacy. www.aacp.org

- *Veterinary Medical School Admission Requirements.* Handbook contains current admissions requirements for the veterinary medical schools in the U.S. and Canada; includes admission data, class profiles. Association of American Veterinary Medical Colleges. www.aavmc.org

- *What Is Public Health?* Brochure providing an overview of public health. Available to students at no cost along with companion brochures, *Reach for Opportunity, for Fulfillment, and for a Career in Public Health* and *You Can Make a Difference, Pursue a Career in Public Health.* Association of Schools of Public Health. www.asph.org

NAAHP Publications

- *Health Professions Admissions Guide: Strategy for Success,* National Association of Advisors for the Health Professions, Inc. (NAAHP). www.naahp.org

- *Write for Success: Preparing a Successful Professional School Application,* National Association of Advisors for the Health Professions, Inc. (NAAHP). www.naahp.org

- *Interviewing for Health Professions Schools,* National Association of Advisors for the Health Professions, Inc. (NAAHP). www.naahp.org

- *Meeting the Challenge of the MCAT: A Test Preparation Guide,* National Association of Advisors for the Health Professions, Inc. (NAAHP). www.naahp.org

Appendix D

Websites for Health Professions Students

HEALTH CAREERS INFORMATION

Allied Health
- American Medical Association, Careers in Allied Health: www.ama-assn.org/ama/no-index/become-member/2322.shtml
- Health Professions Network (HPN): www.healthpronet.org
- Association of Schools of Allied Health Professions (ASAHP): www.asahp.org

Allopathic Medicine
- American Medical Association: www.ama-assn.org

- Association of American Medical Colleges (AAMC) home page — official resource for academic medicine, includes comprehensive information and links: www.aamc.org

- AAMC Tomorrows Doctors — information for those considering medical school: www.aamc.org/students

- Accredited Medical Schools of the U.S. and Canada: services.aamc.org/memberlistings/index.cfm?fuseaction=home.search&search_type=MS

- American Medical Student Association Premed Page: www.amsa.org/premed

- Medical School Admission Test: www.aamc.org/mcat

- Student/Doctor Network Interview Feedback System — reports of medical school applicants about their interview experiences at specific medical schools: www.studentdoctor.net/interview/index.asp

- American Medical College Application Service (AMCAS): www.aamc.org/students/amcas/start.htm

Alternative Medicine
- The American Association of Naturopathic Physicians (AANP): www.naturopathic.org

- American Association of Naturopathic Medical Colleges (AANMC): www.aanmc.org/index.php

- The Naturopathic Medicine Network: www.pandamedicine.com

- National Center for Complementary and Alternative Medicine, National Institutes of Health: www.nccam.nih.gov

- Council of Colleges of Acupuncture and Oriental Medicine: www.ccaom.org

Chiropractic Medicine
- American Chiropractic Association: www.americhiro.org

Dental Medicine
- American Dental Education Association — includes student and applicant information, publications: www.adea.org

- American Dental Association — dental education and career information: www.ada.org

- American Association of Dental Schools Application Service (AADSAS): www.adea.org/dental_education_pathways/aadsas/Pages/default.aspx

Genetic Counseling
- National Society of Genetic Counselors — information on jobs, careers and issues in genetic counseling: www.nsgc.org

- Genetic Counseling Programs — includes international programs, links to resources: www.kumc.edu/gec/prof/gcprogs.html

Health Administration
- Association of University Programs in Health Administration: www.aupha.org

Health Information Science
- American Medical Informatics Association: www.amia.org

Medical Illustration
- Association of Medical Illustrators: www.ami.org

Nursing
- Home page for the American Association of Colleges of Nursing (AACN): www.aacn.nche.edu

- American Academy of Nurse Practitioners: www.aanp.org

- The American College of Nurse-Midwives — information on midwifery education and practice, and related web resources: www.acnm.org

Nutrition
- American Society for Nutrition — listings of graduate programs: www.nutrition.org/education-and-professional-development/graduate-program-directory

Occupational Therapy
- American Occupational /Therapy Association: www.aota.org

Optometry
- Association of Schools and Colleges of Optometry: www.opted.org

Osteopathic Medicine
- American Association of Colleges of Osteopathic Medicine — links to osteopathic medicine schools, can download application material: www.aacom.org

- American Osteopathic Association: www.osteopathic.org

- American Association of Colleges of Osteopathic Medicine Application Service: (AACOMAS): aacomas.aacom.org

Pharmacy
- American Pharmacists Association: www.aphanet.org

- American Association of Colleges of Pharmacy: www.aacp.org

- Pharmacy College Application Service (PharmCAS): www.pharmcas.org

Podiatric Medicine
- American Podiatric Medical Association: www.apma.org

- American Association of Colleges of Podiatric Medicine: www.aacpm.org

- American Association of Colleges of Podiatric Medicine Application Service (AACPMAS): www.e-aacpmas.org

Physical Therapy
- American Physical Therapy Association — links to other sites: www.apta.org

  Physical Therapist Centralized Application Service: www.ptcas.org

Physician Assistant
- American Academy of Physician Assistants: www.aapa.org

- Physician Assistant Education Association: www.paeaonline.org

- Central Application Service for Physician Assistants (CASPA): www.caspaonline.org

Public Health
- American Public Health Association (APHA): largest organization of public health providers in the world; links to science and practice programs, publications, advocacy efforts, news and publications, job resources: www.apha.org

- Association of Schools of Public Health: www.asph.org

- Schools of Public Health Application Service: www.sophas.org

Veterinary Medicine
- NetVet Web — links to hundreds of veterinary sites: netvet.wustl.edu/search.htm

- Association of American Veterinary Colleges: www.aavmc.org

- Veterinary Medical College Application Service: www.aavmc.org/vmcas/vmcas.htm

- American Pre-Veterinary Medical Association: apvma.sdstate.org

- Veterinary Information Network: www.vin.com

- Veterinary Medical College Application Service (VMCAS): aavmc.org/vmcas/vmcas.htm

GENERAL MEDICAL INTERNET RESOURCES

- Explorehealthcareers.org — extensive information on the health professions, summer program listings, articles of interest, particularly geared to minority and disadvantaged students: www.explorehealthcareers.org

- MedWeb Biomedical Internet Resources — large biomedical index of internet resources, comprehensive listing of journals, easy to search: www.medweb.emory.edu/medweb/SPT—Home.php

- MedWorld — Stanford Medical student website, includes selective listing of the best medical sites on the web: www.med.stanford.edu/medworld/home/index_java.html

- Hardin Meta Directory — comprehensive health and medical index sites, directory of health libraries: www.lib.uiowa.edu/hardin/md/idx.html

- PubMed — National Library of Medicine search service to citations in MEDLINE and other databases: www.ncbi.nlm.nih.gov/PubMed

- Health Care Information Resources — extensive listing of health care disciplines and education: hsl.mcmaster.ca/tomflem/disciped.html

POSTBACCALAUREATE PROGRAMS

- NAAHP Information on Postbaccalaureate Premedical Programs — general information on postbac programs: www.naahp.org/resources_Postbac_Article.htm

- AAMC Information on Postbaccalaureate Premedical Programs — comprehensive list of postbac premed programs: services.aamc.org/postbac/index.cfm

HEALTH CARE JOURNALS, CENTERS, ORGANIZATIONS

- Bioethics.net — site of *The American Journal of Bioethics:* www.bioethics.net

- Center for Bioethics, University of Pennsylvania: www.bioethics.upenn.edu

- New England Journal of Medicine — contains abstracts and full text of articles, editorials, letters to editor: www.nejm.org

- American Medical Association — links to advocacy, publications, includes news and past issues from *Journal of American Medical Association*, abstracts from journals: www.ama-assn.org

- Center for Disease Control — links to the separate Institutes, information about grants, education, training: www.cdc.gov

- National Institutes of Health (NIH) — includes links to separate institutes, information about grants: www.nih.gov

INTERNATIONAL HEALTH

- World Health Organization: www.who.int/en

- International Healthcare Opportunities Clearinghouse — listing of health care volunteer opportunities; provides diverse search criteria and links to programs: library.umassmed.edu/ihoc/index.cfm

- Global Health Education Consortium (formerly International Health Medical Education Consortium) — annotated list of websites, related information for those interested in international health: www.globalhealth-ec.org

- International Health Resources — annotated listing of international health sites from UC Berkeley Public Health Library: www.lib.berkeley.edu/PUBL/IntHealth.html

- International Medical Volunteers Association — provides information on how to become international volunteer; links to hundreds of volunteer opportunities: www.imva.org

DISADVANTAGED/MINORITY STUDENT PROGRAMS

- Summer Medical and Dental Education Program (SMDEP): www.smdep.org

- NAAHP Information on Diversity: www.naahp.org/diversity.htm

- NIH Undergraduate Scholarship Program (UGSP): ugsp.nih.gov/home.asp?m=00

- Explore Health Careers: www.explorehealthcareers.org

- AAMC site designed for students underrepresented in medicine: www.aspiringdocs.org

- Premed of Color (Stanford University) resources and links: premedofcolor.org

- National Society for Nontraditional Premedical and Medical Students: www.oldpremeds.org

FINANCIAL AID

- AAMC information on financing your medical education: www.aamc.org/students/financing/start.htm

- The Financial Aid Information Page — includes program to set up personal mailbox for receiving relevant financial aid information: www.finaid.org

- Annual Tuition and Student Fee Reports,for AAMC schools: services.aamc.org/tsfreports

FINDING A PRE-HEALTH ADVISOR

- NAAHP Information on locating the pre-health advisor at your college or university. Also available is an opportunity to find volunteer advisors for students who need one: www.naahp.org/advisors.htm